Multiple Choice Questions
- Anaesthesia

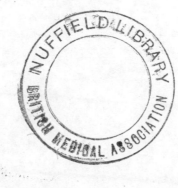

Multiple Choice Questions in Anaesthesia: Basic Sciences

BAKUL KUMAR
MB, BS, DA, FFARCS

Consultant in Anaesthetics and Pain Relief, Dudley Road Hospital, Birmingham

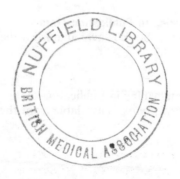

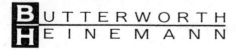

BUTTERWORTH
HEINEMANN

Butterworth-Heinemann Ltd
Linacre House, Jordan Hill, Oxford OX2 8DP

 PART OF REED INTERNATIONAL BOOKS

OXFORD   LONDON   BOSTON
MUNICH   NEW DELHI   SINGAPORE   SYDNEY
TOKYO   TORONTO   WELLINGTON

First published 1992

British Library Cataloguing in Publication Data
A catalogue record for this book is available from the
British Library

Library of Congress Cataloguing in Publication Data
A catalogue record for this book is available from the
Library of Congress

ISBN 0 7506 1556 7

Printed and bound in Great Britain by Biddles Ltd,
Guildford and King's Lynn

Contents

Preface

This book has been compiled as a guide for candidates appearing for FC Anacs. Part 2 examinations. This examination tests the knowledge of the candidate in physiology, pharmacology, statistics, physiological measurement and acid/base. It takes the form of eighty Multiple Choice Questions (MCQ) with equal distribution of questions in physiology and pharmacology with questions in statistics, physiological measurement and acid/base. Each question consists of a stem with five items, the answers of which might be true or false.

The difficulties which arise in answering the MCQs are inadequate preparation of the syllabus and wrong interpretation of the questions. Multiple Choice Questioning is the easiest method by which candidates can be assessed on a variety of subjects in an examination over a short period of time.

I would advise candidates to read standard textbooks and test the knowledge they have gained by attempting MCQs from this book. Correct answers and explanations are given at the back of each set of questions. The bibliography at the end of this book details the books and journals which have been used to compile these MCQs.

Although the book is aimed at candidates preparing for FC Anaes. Part 2 examinations, it will be beneficial for candidates appearing for European Diploma in Anaesthesiology, US FLEX and Board Certification examinations.

Bakul Kumar

Acknowledgements

This book is dedicated to all the trainees who have attended FC Anaes. Part 2 Courses held at Dudley Road Hospital over the last few years and to my wife Corrinne for giving me inspiration to compile this book.

I am grateful to Dr Monica Stokes, Lecturer in Anaesthetics, University of Birmingham, for carefully scrutinizing all the questions and answers and Mrs Christine Hamer of Butterworth-Heinemann for all the encouragement given to me.

1 Central nervous system

1 Isoflurane
A Can trigger malignant hyperpyrexia
B Relaxes the uterus in a dose-dependent manner
C Cough is the commonest side-effect during induction
D Is non-irritant to the airways
E 'Coronary steal phenomenon' has been reported with its use

2 Pharmacokinetics of propofol (Diprivan)
A Extrahepatic mechanisms contribute to its clearance from the blood
B Can be described by a two-compartment model
C Propofol has a large volume of distribution
D Propofol has a low total body clearance
E Propofol has a tendency for slight accumulation

3 Nitrous oxide
A Crosses placental barrier
B Megaloblastic anaemia occurs after 48 hours after its exposure
C Plasma methionine concentration falls by 30% after 8 hours of nitrous oxide administration
D Repeated exposures at intervals of less than 3 days has a cumulative effect
E Abuse can lead to a condition resembling subacute combined degeneration of the spinal cord

Central nervous system: Answers

1 A True
   B True
   C True
   D False
   E True
Isoflurane is fairly pungent and can be an irritant to the upper airways.

2 A True
   B False
   C True
   D True
   E True
Three-compartmental model is used to describe the pharmacokinetic behaviour of propofol (a rapid initial distribution, rapid intermediate phase and a slow final phase). Propofol is highly lipophilic and the initial dilution volume greatly exceeds blood volume. There is extensive redistribution and the steady state volume of distribution is approximately 263 litres.

3 A True
   B False
   C False
   D True
   E True
Megaloblastic anaemia occurs after 6 h exposure in healthy patients and the plasma methionine levels fall to 30% of normal values after 8 h of nitrous oxide

4 Alfentanil
  A Has a low therapeutic index
  B At 5 mcg/kg causes a rise in pulmonary vascular resistance
  C Is one-fifth as potent as fentanyl
  D Causes a decrease in myocardial contractility
  E Hypotension occurs when injected in ASA II to IV patients

5 Opioid receptors
  A Morphine acts on Kappa receptors
  B The effect of stimulation of Sigma receptors is dysphoria and hallucinations
  C Euphoria is due to the stimulation of Delta receptors
  D Nalorphine antagonizes Kappa receptors
  E Pentazocine is a partial agonist

6 Chronic exposure to inhalational anaesthetics can cause:
  A Renal failure
  B Bone marrow depression
  C Immunosuppression
  D Teratogenicity
  E Neurological disease

7 Neuromuscular blockers
  A Suxamethonium releases histamine
  B Vecuronium has a vagolytic effect
  C Alcuronium causes ganglion blockade
  D Gallamine causes vagal stimulation
  E Tubocurare has a sympathomimetic effect

4 A   False
    B   True
    C   False
    D   False
    E   True

Alfentanil has a high therapeutic index (1080) and is one-quarter as potent as fentanyl. It causes an increase in myocardial contractility

5 A   True
    B   True
    C   False
    D   False
    E   True

Morphine acts on Mu and Kappa receptors and euphoria is due to the stimulation of Mu receptors. Nalorphine stimulates Kappa but antagonizes Mu receptors. Pentazocine antagonizes Mu but stimulates Kappa receptors.

6 A   False
    B   True
    C   False
    D   True
    E   True

Acute exposure to inhalational anaesthetics can cause renal failure (methoxyflurane) and immunosuppression.

7 A   True
    B   False
    C   True
    D   False
    E   False

Gallamine and pancuronium are vagolytic and sympathomimetic, whereas suxamethonium causes vagal stimulation.

8 Ethyl alcohol
  A Boiling point is 85°C
  B Is metabolized at the rate of 20 ml/h
  C Follows first-order kinetics
  D Disulfiram inhibits the oxidation of acetyladehyde
  E Is a protein precipitant

9 Droperidol
  A Resembles metoclopramide structurally
  B In low doses is an effective emetic
  C Acts on α-adrenergic receptors
  D Anti-Parkinson drugs treat dystonia caused by droperidol
  E Has a slow onset of action

10 Pharmacokinetics
  A Linear kinetics means rate of elimination of drug is proportionate to the concentration of the drug
  B In zero-order kinetics capacity of enzyme system plays a vital role
  C Plasma clearance is the volume of plasma from which the drug is partially removed per unit time
  D Plasma level of the drug can be measured at zero time
  E Initial decay in the plasma concentration of drug is rapid and called the α phase

11 Drug interactions
  A Monoamine oxidase (MAO) inhibitors interact with pethidine and can cause coma
  B Ecothiopate prolongs suxamethonium block
  C Cigarettes reduce the effect of coumarins
  D Gentamicin interacts with ethacrynic acid causing nephrotoxicity
  E Rifampicin interacts with oral contraceptives

8 A False
   B False
   C True
   D True
   E True
The boiling point of alcohol is 78°C and it metabolizes at a rate of 10 ml/h.

9 A True
   B False
   C True
   D True
   E False
Droperidol is an effective anti-emetic.

10 A True
    B True
    C False
    D False
    E True
Plasma clearance is the volume of plasma from which the drug is completely removed per unit time. It is not possible to measure plasma level of the drug at zero time, so the rate of decay of drug after several minutes is calculated.

11 A True
    B True
    C True
    D False
    E True
Gentamicin interacts with ethacrynic acid causing ototoxicity.

12 Enkephalins
 A Are polypeptides
 B Have the same amino acid squence as β-lipotropin hormone
 C The highest concentration of Met-enkephalin is seen in corpus striatum
 D Released at synaptic opiate receptors facilitate pain signal transmission
 E Produce dependence in man

13 Enflurane
 A Increases cerebral blood flow
 B At 2 MAC (minimum alveolar concentration) depresses systemic arterial pressure by 22%
 C Up to 2–20 ml of 1:100 000 dilution, adrenaline can be safely used during enflurane anaesthesia
 D At 2 MAC increases pulmonary ventilation
 E Less than 3% is metabolized to inorganic fluoride

14 Salicylate poisoning
 A Produces respiratory alkalosis
 B Causes hypofibrinogenaemia
 C Actual bicarbonate is higher than standard bicarbonate
 D There is a negative base excess
 E Hyponatraemia occurs

15 Plasma half-life of:
 A Digoxin is 8 h
 B Insulin is 40 min
 C Curare is 5 min
 D Lignocaine is 90 min
 E Paracetamol is 240 min

12 A False
B True
C True
D False
E False
Enkephalins are pentapeptides which are split off from large endorphins and act as endogenous analgesics.
Met-enkephalin has the same amino acid sequence to residues 61–65 of pituitary hormone β-lipotropin hormone.
Enkephalins released from interneurons inhibit the pain signal. As they are short-acting, dependence in man is not possible.

13 A True
B False
C True
D True
E True
At 1 MAC enflurane depresses the systemic arterial pressure by 22% and at 2 MAC the increase in ventilation is due to a raised P_{CO_2}.

14 A True
B True
C False
D True
E False
Respiratory alkalosis is seen initially. A negative base excess indicates metabolic acidosis and hypernatraemia seen is due to water loss.

15 A False
B True
C False
D True
E True
The plasma half-life of digoxin is 48 h and of curare is 12 min.

16 Apparent volume of distribution
A Is the fluid volume which would contain the known dose of drug administered in a uniform plasma concentration
B Of insulin is 50
C Of frusemide is 20
D Of aspirin is 12
E Of digoxin is 500

17 Etomidate
A Is an imidazole derivative
B Its metabolites are conjugated to form glucuronide compounds
C Decreases the intraocular pressure
D The total volume of distribution is large
E Liver blood flow does not affect clearance

18 Thiopentone
A Between 50 and 60% is reversibly bound to albumin
B Elimination half-life is between 5 and 12 h
C Total apparent volume of distribution is between 1.4 and 2.3 l/kg body weight
D Ionized thiopentone is soluble in lipids and thus pharmacologically inactive
E Has a pK_a of 7.6

19 Physical properties of volatile anaesthetic agents
A Halothane has an oil/gas partition coefficient of 236
B Minimum alveolar concentration of isoflurane is 1.7
C Molecular weight of enflurane is 184
D Isoflurane has a blood/gas partition coefficient of 13.0
E The oil/gas partition coefficients of enflurane and isoflurane are similar

16 A True
    B True
    C False
    D True
    E True
The apparent volume of distribution of frusemide is 7. The higher the volume of distribution, the chances of dialysis becoming effective become less.

17 A True
    B True
    C True
    D False
    E False
Interestingly, in spite of cardiovascular stability, etomidate has been shown to cause a fall in intraocular pressure. Etomidate has a high hepatic extraction ratio, and a fall in liver blood flow affects clearance

18 A False
    B True
    C True
    D False
    E True
Around 75–85% of thiopentone is reversibly bound to albumin and the ionized thiopentone is insoluble in lipids.
pK_a is the negative logarithm of the dissociation constant.

19 A True
    B False
    C True
    D False
    E True
Isoflurane has a MAC of 1.2 as compared with 1.7 of enflurane and a blood gas partition coefficient of 1.4 as compared with 13.0 of methoxyflurane.

20 Atracurium
  A Is a monquaternary ammonium salt
  B Is destroyed by the enzymatic hydrolysis of the ester grouping
  C Has a shelf-life of 3 years when stored in a refrigerator
  D Acidity accelerates its decomposition
  E Has no vagolytic activity

21 Sodium valproate
  A Is a branched-chain liquid fatty acid
  B Is effective in grand mal seizures
  C Takes 3 weeks for the effect to develop
  D Interferes with platelet aggregation
  E Is metabolized by hepatic microsomal systems

22 In patients with glaucoma, the following conditions affect the intraocular pressure
  A An increased intensity of light
  B Carbonic anhydrase inhibitors
  C A diet high in vitamin A
  D Parasympathetic blockade with atropine
  E An increased pressure on the jugular vein

23 Phenytoin
  A Has a half-life of 22 h
  B Absorption is rapid by the IM or IV route
  C Is used to treat cardiac arrhythmias
  D Can cause megaloblastic anaemia due to vitamin B12 deficiency
  E Long-term use does not alter thyroid function

20 A False
  B True
  C False
  D False
  E True
Atracurium is a bis quaternary ammonium salt which in addition
to Hoffman degradation is also destroyed by enzymatic hydrolysis.
It has a shelf-life of 2 years and alkalinity accelerates the
decomposition of atracurium.

21 A True
  B False
  C False
  D True
  E True
Sodium valproate is effective in petit mal and mixed seizures and is
effective within 14 days after commencing therapy.

22 A False
  B True
  C False
  D True
  E True
Intensity of light has no definite effect on the intraocular pressure
(IOP). Carbonic anhydrase inhibitors, like acetazolamide, decrease
the IOP by decreasing the movement of water and electrolytes in
the aqueous humour. A pressure on the jugular vein decreases the
hydrostatic pressure at the corneoscleral junction, thus increasing
the absorption of intraocular fluid.

23 A True
  B False
  C True
  D False
  E True
The absorption of phenytoin is effective only when given IV and
orally. It causes macrocytosis and megaloblastic anaemia due to
folic acid deficiency. Long-term use gives falsely low thyroid
function tests.

24 Lignocaine
A Is an amide
B Is excreted unchanged
C In overdose, death occurs due to ventricular fibrillation
D Is absorbed relatively slowly from the gastrointestinal tract
E Is insoluble in water

25 Narcotic antagonists
A Levallorphan is an N-allyl derivative of levorphanol
B Naloxone has a morphine-like action
C Nalorphine is a pure antagonist
D Pentazocine has an agonist–antagonist action
E Pentazocine can be used to reverse the respiratory depression caused by fentanyl

26 Levodopa
A Is structurally related to apomorphine
B Crosses the blood/brain barrier when administered orally
C Causes increased vigour and a sense of well-being
D Causes hypertension
E Acts by replenishing deficient stores of dopamine in the cortex

24 A True
    B False
    C True
    D False
    E False
Lignocaine is metabolized in the liver to xylidide and
methylglycine. It is absorbed equally from the gastrointestinal tract
and after parenteral administration.

25 A True
    B False
    C False
    D True
    E True
Nalorphine possesses some morphine-like action. The technique
called 'sequential analgesia' consists of use of a high dose of
fentanyl in the intraoperative period and reversing the respiratory
depression caused by it at the end of the surgery with pentazocine
or nalbuphine.

26 A True
    B False
    C True
    D False
    E False
Levodopa, in addition to being structurally similar to
apomorphine, shares the same pharmacological properties such as
causing nausea and vomiting by acting on the chemoreceptor
trigger zone. When given orally, 95% of the dose is decarboxylated
peripherally to dopamine which does not cross the blood/brain
barrier. Therapeutic doses cause orthostatic hypotension in normal
subjects and patients with Parkinson's disease. It acts by
replenishing dopamine stores in the corpus striatum.

27 Toxicity of drugs
   A LD50 is that dose which kills 50% of animals under stated conditions
   B In a chronic toxicity study the drug is given to animals of a single species for 30 days
   C ED50 is the mean effective index
   D The ratio of LD50 to ED50 is calculated as the therapeutic index
   E To check the effect of a drug during the childbearing period, during trials, the drug is fed to female rats before first mating

28 Drugs and lipid solubility
   A Is influenced by the presence of an ionizable group
   B Unionized drug is non-diffusible
   C Environmental pH has no action
   D Buprenorphine is lipid soluble
   E A part of the prolonged action of intrathecal morphine is due to its lipid solubility

29 Drug interactions
   A Phenytoin displaces thyroxine from its carrier protein
   B Warfarin is displaced by nalidixic acid
   C Fatty acids do not influence the binding of phenylbutazone to albumin
   D Occurs when two drugs have affinity for separate binding sites
   E Sulphonamides displace bilirubin and cause kernicterus

30 Barbiturates
   A Decrease the venous return
   B With long half-life are highly protein bound
   C Excretion can be enhanced by making the urine acidic
   D The action of barbitone is potentiated in hepatic failure
   E Cause diarrhoea

27 A True
    B False
    C False
    D True
    E False
In chronic toxicity studies the drug is given to animals of two
species for 90 days. ED50 is the median effective index. To check
the effect of drug during the childbearing period, the drug is given
to both male and female rats prior to mating and extending
through production of two litters.

28 A True
    B False
    C False
    D True
    E True
The un-ionized drug is diffusible across a membrane.

29 A True
    B True
    C False
    D False
    E True

30 A True
    B False
    C False
    D False
    E False
Barbiturates with short half-lives are highly protein bound and
their excretion can be enhanced by alkalinizing the urine.
Barbitone is metabolized and excreted by the kidneys, hence its
action is not potentiated in patients with hepatic failure.

31 Methadone
  A Causes hypoglycaemia
  B Causes biliary tract spasm
  C Can cause peripheral vasodilatation
  D Is poorly absorbed from the stomach
  E Amount of methadone excreted in the urine is increased when the urine is alkaline

32 Pethidine
  A Is structurally related to atropine
  B Onset of analgesic activity after IM injection is 35 minutes
  C In equianalgesic doses pethidine and morphine produce equal amount of sedation
  D Respiratory depression caused by it can be antagonized by nalorphine
  E About 60% is bound to plasma proteins

33 Morphine
  A Causes dysphoria
  B Causes venodilatation
  C Causes miosis by acting on the Edinger Westphal nucleus
  D Relaxes the ureters
  E Is potentiated by neostigmine

34 Plasma half-life of:
  A Digoxin is 40 min
  B Lignocaine is 90 min
  C Glyceryl trinitrate is 60 min
  D Insulin is 40 min
  E Paracetamol is 240 min

31 A False
    B True
    C True
    D False
    E False
Methadone is well absorbed from the stomach and can be detected
in plasma within 30 min of oral ingestion. A major side-effect is
hyperglycaemia and the amount of methadone excreted in the
urine can be increased by making the urine acidic.

32 A True
    B False
    C False
    D True
    E False
The onset of analgesic activity following IM injection is within
10 min and about 40% of the drug is bound to plasma proteins
and is chiefly metabolized in the liver. In equi-analgesic doses
pethidine produces less sedation than morphine.

33 A True
    B True
    C True
    D False
    E True

34 A False
    B True
    C False
    D True
    E True
The plasma half-life of digoxin is 48 h and that of glyceryl trinitrate
is 35 min.

35 Isoflurane
  A Is a monomer of enflurane
  B Produces a dose-related increase in the total peripheral resistance
  C Increases respiratory rate and decreases tidal volume
  D At 1 MAC concentration has no effect on cerebral oxygen consumption
  E Less than 0.5% inhaled isoflurane is recovered as urinary metabolites

36 Phenytoin
  A Absorption after oral administration is rapid
  B Is 80–95% bound to plasma proteins
  C Its concentration in the cerebrospinal fluid is equal to the unbound fraction in plasma
  D Toxic doses cause sluggish tendon reflexes
  E Causes glycosuria

37 Methadone
  A Is well absorbed from the stomach
  B Has a long duration of action
  C Propoxyphene is an analogue of methadone
  D Is available in laevorotatory form
  E Therapeutic effect lasts for 12 h

35 A False
B False
C True
D False
E True
Isoflurane is a dimer of enflurane and it produces a dose-related decrease in the peripheral resistance. At 1 MAC concentration it decreases the cerebral oxygen consumption.

36 A False
B True
C True
D False
E True
The absorption of phenytoins after oral administration is slow, variable and occasionally incomplete. They are mainly bound to albumin and its apparent volume of distribution is about 70% of body weight and could be seven times larger if calculated on the basis of unbound drug. When toxic doses are reached, it causes blurred vision, mydriasis and hyperactive tendon reflexes. Phenytoin causes hyperglycaemia and glycosuria due to the inhibition of insulin secretion.

37 A False
B True
C True
D False
E False
Methadone is well absorbed from the intestine. Propoxyphene is an ester as compared with methadone which is a ketone. Methadone is available as a racemic mixture. Methadone is effective for 6 h.

38 Cocaine
  A   In small doses causes bradycardia
  B   Has a direct action on the heat-regulating centre
  C   Is fairly effective when given orally
  D   Is less toxic after subcutaneous injection
  E   Interferes with the uptake of noradrenaline by the adrenergic nerve terminals

39 Ethyl alcohol
  A   Is rapidly absorbed by diffusion in the gastrointestinal tract
  B   Rate of metabolism of alcohol is independent of dehydrogenase system
  C   Causes a rise in cerebral blood flow
  D   High doses cause tachycardia
  E   Can cause sodium retention

40 Monoamine oxidase inhibitors (MAOI)
  A   Reduce cardiac output
  B   Cause euphoria and respiratory stimulation
  C   Tranylcypromine can cause hypotension
  D   Hypertensive crisis occurs if patients on MAOI ingest tyramine-containing foods
  E   Effect is terminated after discontinuation of medication

38 A True
   B True
   C False
   D False
   E True

Cocaine is ineffective when given orally because it is hydrolysed in the gastrointestinal tract. It causes bradycardia due to vagal stimulation in small doses. The onset of 'cocaine fever' is preceded by a chill which indicates that the body is adjusting its temperature to a higher level. After subcutaneous injection, cocaine remains in the body for a long time because of slow destruction, thus causing the side-effects.

39 A True
   B False
   C False
   D False
   E True

Alcohol has no effect on the cerebral blood flow. In low doses it causes a rise in heart rate and stroke volume, but in high doses alcohol produces bradycardia. It causes sodium retention initially by suppressing antidiuretic hormone and producing diuresis. The conversion of alcohol to acetaldehyde reaches a maximum when the dehydrogenase system is saturated.

40 A True
   B True
   C True
   D True
   E False

MAOI reduces the cardiac output by blocking the sympathetic system. Its action persists long after elimination or discontinuation of the drug. Tranylcypromine can cause postural hypotension and potentiate other hypotensive agents.

41 Hypnotics
A Chloral hydrate is rapidly metabolized in the red blood cells (RBCs), kidney and liver
B Promethazine acts on H1 receptor
C Paraldehyde is partly excreted unchanged by the lungs
D Chlormethiazole is related to vitamin B6
E Half-life of chlormethiazole is 4 h

42 Vecuronium
A Has a bisquaternary structure
B 20% of it is excreted via the kidneys
C Its volume of distribution is four times that of pancuronium
D Children are more resistant to its effects than adults
E Block is potentiated more with halothane than with isoflurane

43 Toxicity due to local anaesthetics
A Plain bupivacaine is safe at 2–3 mg/kg body weight over a 4 h period
B Convulsions are seen when the dose of plain lignocaine reaches 15 mg/kg
C Bupivacaine increases arrhythmogenic threshold to adrenaline
D Etidocaine can cause ventricular tachycardia
E Electromechanical dissociation is a common side-effect of cocaine toxicity

44 Paracetamol
A Is a metabolite of phenacetin
B Causes methaemoglobinaemia
C Causes dose-dependent hepatic necrosis
D Its metabolite is activated by glutathione
E N-Acetylcysteine is helpful in the treatment of paracetamol poisoning

41 A True
   B True
   C True
   D False
   E False
Chlormethiazole is related to vitamin B1 (thiamine) and has a half-life of 50 min.

42 A False
   B True
   C True
   D True
   E False
Vecuronium is a monoquaternary structure of which 20% is excreted via the kidneys and 12% in the bile in the first 24 hours. Its block is potentiated more by isoflurane than by halothane.

43 A True
   B False
   C True
   D True
   E False
Convulsions are seen when the dose of plain lignocaine reaches between 5 and 10 mg/kg body weight. The toxic side-effect of cocaine is ventricular fibrillation.

44 A True
   B False
   C False
   D False
   E True
Phenacetin (and not paracetamol) causes methaemoglobinaemia. Paracetamol causes dose-dependent hepatic necrosis, and its metabolite, an *N*-hydroxy derivative, is inactivated by glutathione. *N*-Acetylcysteine is rich in sulphydryl groups which aid the production of liver glutathione.

45 Drug–receptor combination
A   Covalent bonding is highly stable
B   Van der Waal's forces are weak bonds
C   Hydrogen bonds have a strength of 2–7 kcal/mol
D   α-adrenergic blockers share Van der Waal's forces
E   Van der Waal's forces represent long-range attractive forces

46 Ketamine
A   Causes transient apnoea
B   Causes a fall in intraocular pressure
C   Resembles haloperidol in action on α- and β-receptors
D   Shows dominant alpha rhythm in EEG
E   4-Aminopyridine shortens the period of sleep

47 Drug metabolism
A   Amphetamine breaks down by oxidation
B   Amine group of local anaesthetics break down by reduction
C   Microsomal enzymes help break down pethidine
D   Morphine undergoes glucuronidation
E   Sulphonamides undergo acetylation

48 Chlormethazole
A   Has anti-emetic properties
B   Causes bradycardia
C   Is available as 0.6% solution in 5% dextrose
D   Is beneficial in stabilizing alcohol-free regimen
E   Can be effective in status asthmaticus

45 A True
   B True
   C True
   D False
   E False
Covalent bonding is highly stable and the prolonged action of adrenergic blocks seen is due to irreversible binding of the drug to the receptors. Van der Waal's forces are weak bonds and represent short-range attractive forces.

46 A True
   B False
   C True
   D False
   E True
Ketamine raises the intraocular and intracranial pressure and in the EEG shows absent alpha rhythm and a dominant theta activity.

47 A True
   B False
   C True
   D True
   E True
Amide group of local anaesthetics break down by hydrolysis.

48 A True
   B False
   C False
   D True
   E False
A 0.8% solution in 4% dextrose is available which is used to control status epilepticus (and not asthmaticus), delerium and tremors.

49 Minimum alveolar concentration (MAC) of isoflurane
A   Lies halfway between the MAC of halothane and enflurane in middle-aged adults
B   10% of nitrous oxide is equivalent to 0.2% of isoflurane
C   Increases with age
D   Is decreased in hypothermia
E   Is unchanged during pregnancy

50 Propofol (Divprivan)
A   Has no effect on whole blood clotting time
B   Pre-treatment with alcohol on the day of anaesthesia potentiates propofol anaesthesia
C   Has a similar therapeutic ratio to thiopentone
D   Shows a central anticholinergic effect
E   Pre-medication with papaveretum increases propofol-induced sleeping time

51 Midazolam
A   In plasma exists as a free acid
B   Initial fall in plasma concentration is due to rapid distribution
C   The principal metabolite is α-hydroxymidazolam
D   Bioavailability following IM injection is 90%
E   In elderly patients (62–76 years of age), 0.2 mg/kg induces sleep in all cases

49 A True
B False
C False
D True
E False
The MAC of isoflurane is 1.15, halothane 0.75 and enflurane 1.68.
Nitrous oxide with a MAC of 104 at 1 atmosphere decreases the
MAC of isoflurane and 10% nitrous oxide is equivalent to 0.1% of
isoflurane. The MAC of isoflurane decreases with age and during
pregnancy and hypothermia.

50 A True
B False
C True
D False
E True
Unlike thiopentone, pre-treatment with alcohol on the day of
anaesthesia does not potentiate propofol anaesthesia.

51 A False
B True
C True
D True
E False
Midazolam is a free base which is lipid soluble. After an IV
injection the plasma concentration falls by 10% within 1 h due to
rapid distribution. The principal metabolite of midazolam has a
shorter half-life than the parent drug (1.5 h). A dose of 0.2 mg/kg
produces sleep in only 70% of cases as compared with 0.3 mg/kg
which produces sleep in all cases.

52 Levodopa and drug interactions
A In the presence of MAO inhibitors, hypertension occurs
B Tricyclic antidepressants potentiate the effects of levodopa
C Intravenous physostigmine exacerbate Parkinsonian symptoms in the presence of levodopa
D Pyridoxine reverses the therapeutic effect of levodopa
E Reserpine potentiates the action of levodopa

53 Pentazocine
A Is a partial agonist
B Has half the potency of morphine
C Is used for sequential analgesia
D Can cause bradycardia and euphoria
E Is broken down in the kidney

54 Benzodiazepines
A Diazepam is rapidly absorbed when administered orally or IV
B Diazepam is eliminated in a triphasic pattern
C Side-effects include psychoses and sudden suicidal impulses
D Cigarette smoking increases their effectiveness
E Diazepam when given to mothers causes hypotonia and hyperthermia in neonates

55 Physostigmine
A Is a quaternary amine
B The usual dose is 0.5–1.0 mg IV
C Can reverse psychotomimetic effects caused by ketamine
D Is excreted mainly by the kidneys
E Increases the peristalitic activity in ureters

52 A True
B False
C False
D True
E True

As MAOI interact with levodopa, the MAOI should be stopped at least 14–30 days before the initiation of levodopa. Tricyclics diminish the effect of levodopa by producing extrapyramidal side-effects. Physostigmine exacerbates symptoms in untreated patients with Parkinson's disease by enhancing the cholinergic transmission in the extrapyramidal system. Reserpine potentiates the action of levodopa by depleting the central dopamine stores.

53 A True
B False
C True
D False
E False

Pentazocine is one-third more potent than morphine and it causes tachycardia and dysphoria. It is metabolized in the liver.

54 A True
B False
C True
D False
E False

Diazepam is eliminated in a biphasic manner, with a rapid phase ($t_{\frac{1}{2}}$ of 2–3 h), followed by a slow decay with a half-life of 3–8 days. When it is administered to mothers, diazepam causes hypotonia and hypothermia in neonates.

55 A False
B True
C True
D False
E True

Physostigmine is a tertiary amine which crosses the blood/brain barrier thus reversing the psychotomimetic effects of ketamine. It is mainly metabolized in the liver by hydrolytic cleavage at the ester linkage by cholinesterases.

56 Methohexitone
A   Is ionized in solution with a pK_a of 8.1
B   Has a distribution half-life of 5.6 min
C   Total volume of distribution is 0.8 l/kg
D   Around 70–75% is bound to the plasma proteins
E   Hepatic blood flow has no effect on its metabolism

57   Phenothiazines
A   Have atropine-like actions in high doses
B   Can intensify vasodilatation
C   Cause a fall in body temperature
D   Cause shortening of P-R interval
E   Dystonias occur in the elderly patients

58 Salicylates
A   Alleviate pain by acting on the peripheral nervous system
B   Augment heat dissipation
C   Have a choleretic effect
D   Prolong bleeding time due to hypoprothrombinaemia
E   Cross the placental barrier easily

56 A   False
   B   True
   C   False
   D   True
   E   False
Methohexitone is ionized in solution with a pK_a of 7.9 and its total volume of distribution lies between 1.1 and 2.2 l/kg.

57 A   True
   B   True
   C   True
   D   False
   E   False
Phenothiazines intensify vasodilatation due to their alpha-adrenergic blocking effect. Although they cause a fall in core temperature, the extremities are warm due to vasodilatation. Phenothiazines cause prolonged PR and QRS intervals due to slowed conduction. Dystonia is a side-effect in children and young adults.

58 A   False
   B   True
   C   True
   D   False
   E   True
Salicylates act peripherally on the prostaglandin system and centrally on the hypothalamus. They augment heat dissipation by increasing the peripheral blood flow and sweating. Salicylates increase the volume output of bile but decrease the total cholate excretion. They prolong bleeding time by blocking the adhesion of platelets to the connective tissue or collagen fibres.

59 Thiopentone sodium
A Is a sulphur analogue of pentobarbitone
B 'Acute tolerance' is seen due to rapid bolus injection
C Increased binding occurs in malnutrition
D Breakdown products are excreted by kidneys and gastrointestinal tract
E Causes a rise in oxygen consumption

60 Neuromuscular blockers
A Metabolic alkalosis potentiates curare
B Respiratory alkalosis potentiates vecuronium
C Hypokalaemia prolongs the action of pancuronium
D Hypothermia prolongs the action of atracurium
E Frusemide potentiates the action of curare

61 Ideal local anaesthetic drug should:
A Have a long latency period
B Be water soluble
C Cause excitation before blocking
D Be autoclavable
E Be used with a vasoconstrictor

62 Diazepam
A Has propylene glycol as the solvent
B Acts on the limbic system
C Causes tachycardia
D Decreases MAC of halothane by 20%
E Causes a fall in $PaCO_2$

59 A True
    B True
    C False
    D True
    E False
Thiopentone, when injected rapidly, causes consciousness to return at a higher plasma level than the same dose if injected slowly ('acute tolerance'). It causes a fall in oxygen consumption and has a decreased protein binding in malnutrition due to hypoproteinaemia.

60 A True
    B False
    C True
    D True
    E True
The action of curare and pancuronium is potentiated by metabolic alkalosis and the action of all neuromuscular blockers in the presence of hypokalaemia and diuretics is potentiated. The action of vecuronium is potentiated by respiratory acidosis and the action of atracurium is prolonged in hypothermic patients because the breakdown of atracurium is temperature dependent.

61 A False
    B True
    C False
    D True
    E False
An ideal local anaesthetic drug should have a short latency period and should not cause excitation before blocking.

62 A True
    B True
    C True
    D False
    E False
The solvent in diazemuls is soyabean oil and diazepam decreases the MAC of halothane by 35% and with large doses there is a rise in $PaCO_2$.

63 Dantrolene
 A Acts by increasing the amount of calcium released from the sarcoplasmic reticulum
 B Depresses polysynaptic reflexes
 C Mean half-life is 9 h
 D Causes euphoria and light-headedness
 E Is effective in athetoid cerebral palsy

64 Tricyclic antidepressants
 A Become effective in 2–3 weeks after starting treatment
 B Have a weak anticholinergic effect
 C Cause bradycardia
 D Imipramine causes inversion or flattening of the T waves
 E Hyperventilation is seen in amitryptyline poisoning

65 Phenytoin sodium
 A Stabilizes excitable cell membranes
 B Is metabolized by rhodanase
 C Can cause nystagmus
 D Wide-set eyes, broad jaw and finger deformities sum up fetal-hydantoin syndrome
 E Is specific in the treatment of digitalis-induced dysrrhythmias

66 Sufentanil
 A Is a thienyl derivative of fentanyl
 B Distributes slowly to certain tissues like fat
 C Is twice as potent as fentanyl
 D Causes a fall in systolic blood pressure
 E Its haemodynamic response is age-related

63 A False
    B False
    C True
    D True
    E True
Dantrolene acts by decreasing the amount of calcium released from the sarcoplasmic reticulum. It does not depress polysynaptic reflexes, unlike the centrally acting muscle relaxants such as mephensin. It is effective in the treatment of malignant hyperpyrexia, cerebral palsy, multiple sclerosis and muscle spasms associated with paraplegia.

64 A True
    B False
    C False
    D True
    E False
As opposed to phenothiazines, tricyclics are potent anticholinergic agents. They cause tachycardia and all the adverse effects are due to blockade of uptake of catecholamines. In amitryptyline overdose there is respiratory depression.

65 A True
    B False
    C True
    D True
    E True
Phenytoin sodium is metabolized by hepatic microsomal enzymes.

66 A True
    B False
    C False
    D True
    E True
Sufentanil distributes rapidly and extensively to all tissues and is 5 to 10 times more potent than fentanyl. The fall in blood pressure caused by sufentanil depends on the age of the patient.

67 Parasympathomimetics
A Bethanechol is useful in relieving urinary retention
B Cause a rise in blood pressure
C Acetylcholine dilates coronary vessels
D Acetylcholine prolongs the effective refractory period in the atrial muscle
E Carbachol produces increased gastrointestinal activity associated with minimal cardiovascular effects

68 Drug interactions
A Ranitidine reduces bupivacaine clearance
B Prenylamine precipitates A–V block in the presence of lignocaine
C Pethidine increases lignocaine-induced convulsions
D Adrenaline can provoke myocardial depression due to bupivacaine
E Acidosis enhances lignocaine toxicity

69 Chlorpromazine produces:
A Sedation
B Suppression of abnormal behaviour in schizophrenia
C Elevation of mood in endogenous depression
D Suppression of vomiting due to morphine
E Suppression of symptoms of the alcohol withdrawal syndrome

67 A True
    B False
    C True
    D False
    E True
Bethanechol is effective in relieving urinary retention (post-operative and post-partum) in the absence of mechanical obstruction. Hypertensive patients react to parasympathomimetics with a precipitous fall in blood pressure and an overdose may cause cardiac arrest. Acetylcholine essentially causes vasodilatation of all vascular beds. It also decreases the strength of contraction, slows the rate of conduction of the action potential and shortens the duration of action potential and effective refractory period. Acetylcholine and methacholine induce relatively marked cardiovascular effects, whereas drugs such as carbachol and bethanechol produce increased tone, peristaltic activity with minimal cardiovascular effects.

68 A False
    B True
    C True
    D False
    E True
Lignocaine clearance is diminished by cimetidine and propranolol. Prenylamine, a catechol-depleting agent which is used in the treatment of angina, can precipitate A–V block in the presence of lignocaine. Pethidine increases lignocaine-induced convulsions, possibly because norpethidine, its metabolite, is a convulsant. Adrenaline prevents the myocardial depression caused by bupivacaine.

69 A False
    B True
    C True
    D True
    E False

70 **Organophosphorous compounds**
   A   Cause hypoglycaemia
   B   Muscle fasciculation precedes paralysis
   C   Cause drying of secretions
   D   Cause miosis
   E   Cause bradycardia and sweating

71 **Chloral derivatives (e.g. chloral hydrate and triclofos)**
   A   Have analgesic activity
   B   Do not affect blood pressure
   C   Chloral hydrate is reduced to trichlorethanol
   D   Cause 'hangover' effect
   E   Causes scarlatiniform rash

72 **Lithium**
   A   Mimics extracellular sodium and potassium ions
   B   Is absorbed from the gastrointestinal tract
   C   Passes the blood/brain barrier easily
   D   Is reabsorbed in the distal convoluted tubule
   E   Has insulin-like action

70 A False
B True
C False
D True
E True
Organophosphorous compounds cause hyperglycaemia, copious bronchial secretions, hypoxia and pulmonary oedema. The treatment of overdose consists of gastric lavage and atropine to reverse muscarinic effects.

71 A False
B True
C True
D False
E True
Chloral hydrate derivatives, like barbiturates, cause excitement or delerium in the presence of pain. Allergic reactions to chloral derivatives include erythema, urticaria, scarlatiniform rash.

72 A False
B True
C False
D False
E True
Lithium mimicks extracellular sodium and intracellular potassium. It is reabsorbed in the proximal convoluted tubule uninfluenced by the diuretics. Lithium causes an increase in skeletal muscle glycogen accompanied by severe depletion of glycogen from the liver.

73 Pethidine
- A Pethidine (100 mg) parenterally is equal to 15 mg of morphine
- B Causes tremors and seizures
- C Causes pupillary dilatation
- D Increases the sensitivity of labyrinthine apparatus
- E Inhibits the release of antidiuretic hormone (ADH)

74 Propoxyphene
- A Its analgesic activity lies in the laevo isomer
- B Is structurally related to methadone
- C Causes mild euphoria
- D Half-life following IV route is twice that following oral dose
- E In toxic doses causes convulsions

75 Anticholinesterases
- A Physostigmine is obtained from calabar bean
- B Edrophonium has a long duration of action
- C Inhibit the acetylcholinesterase enzymes
- D Physostigmine stimulates autonomic ganglia
- E Causes a fall in reabsorption of aqueous humour

73 A False
B True
C False
D True
E False

100 mg of pethidine is equal to 10 mg of morphine with regard to potency. Toxic doses cause excitation-like tremors, muscle twitches and seizures. It causes pupillary constriction like any other narcotics. As the sensitivity of labryinthine apparatus is increased by pethidine, a higher incidence of nausea and vomiting is seen when given to ambulant patients. Pethidine causes the release of ADH, stimulation of chemoreceptor trigger zone, inhibition of adrenocorticotropin (ACTH) and gonadotrophic hormones.

74 A False
B True
C True
D False
E True

The analgesic activity of propoxyphene is due to its dextro isomer (dextropropoxyphene), whereas the laevo isomer has antitussive action. The mean half-life following an oral dose is 14.6 h which is higher than the value obtained after IV injection.

75 A True
B False
C True
D False
E False

Calabar bean from which physostigmine is derived is the dried ripe seed of *Physostigma venenosum*. Edrophonium has an extremely brief duration of action and is used in the diagnosis and treatment of myasthenia gravis. The anticholinesterases inhibit the enzymes at the site of cholinergic transmission, with consequent accumulation and action of endogenous acetylcholine liberated both by cholinergic impulses and smaller amounts by continual leakage during the resting stage. At high doses, physostigmine blocks the effects of autonomic ganglia. Anticholinesterases produce a fall in the intraocular pressure as a result of facilitation of reabsorption of aqueous humour.

76 Drugs and the autonomic nervous system
   A   Reserpine accumulates noradrenaline at extracellular sites
   B   Guanethedine depletes noradrenaline at adrenergic nerve
        endings
   C   Phenoxybenzamine locks the endogenous transmitter at the
        post-synaptic receptor
   D   Physostigmine is a cholinergic blocker
   E   Tranylcypromine potentiates the effects of catecholamines

77 Narcotic antagonists
   A   Nalorphine induces antidiuretic effect
   B   Naloxone is one-fifth as potent as nalorphine
   C   Naloxone precipitates a withdrawal syndrome after chronic
        doses of pentazocine
   D   Naloxone is metabolized and excreted by the kidneys
   E   Naloxone is one-fifth as potent when given orally as compared
        with parenteral administration

76 A False
 B True
 C True
 D False
 E False
Reserpine destroys noradrenaline by mitochondrial MAO and depletes them from adrenergic nerve endings. Physostigmine is a cholinomimetic and acts by inhibition of enzymatic breakdown of acetylcholine. Tranylcypromine is a MAO inhibitor which potentiates the effect of tyramine.

77 A False
 B False
 C True
 D False
 E False
Nalorphine antagonizes the antidiuretic effect caused by morphine. Nalorphine is one-seventh as potent as naloxone in precipitating withdrawal symptoms in morphine-dependent people. Naloxone is absorbed and metabolized very rapidly in its first passage through the liver and is only one-fiftieth as potent when given orally. The doses of naloxone required to precipitate withdrawals after pentazocine administration are very high as compared with those used for morphine.

78 Local anaesthetics
A Maximum topical dose for cocaine is 400 mg
B Maximum safety dose for procaine is 1000 mg
C Maximum dose for bupivacaine is 3 mg/kg body weight
D Prilocaine is highly effective when used topically
E A 2–4% strength of lignocaine is used for topical analgesia

79 Carbimazole
A Selectively blocks the incorporation of iodine into organic molecules
B Is useful in the treatment of hyperthyroidism
C Selectively blocks iodide uptake by thyroid gland
D Decreases basal metabolic rate
E Can produce goitre by increased secretion of thyrotropin

78 A False
   B True
   C True
   D False
   E True

Local anaesthetics once absorbed into the circulation can cause
systemic toxicity and in particular affecting the cardiovascular and
central nervous system. Toxic blood concentrations can cause
convulsions followed by respiratory depression, coma and
cardiovascular collapse. The treatment of toxic reactions includes
airway management and oxygenation. Convulsions may be treated
with diazepam or thiopentone.
The maximum safe dose is that quoted for regional blocks and if
the same dose is injected intravenously can cause serious toxicity.
The maximum safe dosages are as follows: cocaine 3 mg/kg;
bupivacaine 150 mg without adrenaline and 200 mg with adrenaline
(2 mg/kg); lignocaine 200–400 mg without adrenaline (3 mg/kg) and
500 mg with adrenaline (7 mg/kg); chlorprocaine 1000 mg with
adrenaline and 800 mg without adrenaline; prilocaine 600 mg with
adrenaline and 400 mg without adrenaline.
Cocaine is used for surface anaesthesia; a 4–5% concentration is
recommended for mucous membranes of the nose, mouth and
throat.

79 A False
   B True
   C True
   D False
   E False

Carbimazole is an imidazoline derivative. It is used in the
treatment of hyperthyroidism. Carbimazole prevents the oxidation
of iodine and inhibits coupling of iodotyrosines to form
iodothyronines, thus inhibiting the formation of thyroxine. It is
metabolized in the thyroid gland and a majority of it is excreted in
the urine. The initial dose is 20–60 mg/day.

80 Anticholinergics
  A   Quaternary ammonium compounds are lipid soluble
  B   Cause cycloplegia
  C   Inhibit gastric acid secretion
  D   Are used in the treatment of glaucoma
  E   Constrict the oesophageal sphincter

81 Tricyclic antidepressants
  A   Cause mood elevation in a normal subject
  B   Can be used as sedatives
  C   Have a significant effect on dopaminergic receptors
  D   Cause urinary incontinence
  E   Lower the blood pressure

82 Opium alkaloids
  A   Codeine is an ethylmorphine
  B   Heroin is derived from morphine following deacetylation
  C   Thebaine has hydroxyl groups which are methylated
  D   Papaverine has morphine-like effects
  E   Noscapine belongs to benzylisoquinoline class of alkaloids

80 A False
   B True
   C False
   D False
   E False

Anticholinergics are lipid insoluble and hence do not cross the blood/brain barrier. They cause difficulty in accommodation (cycloplegia) and can exacerbate glaucoma and urinary retention in the elderly. Anticholinergics relax the oesophageal sphincters and hence should be avoided in patients with symptomatic reflux.

81 A False
   B True
   C False
   D False
   E True

Unlike MAO inhibitors, tricyclics do not cause mood elevation in normal subjects. Tricyclics have no effect on dopamine receptors (unlike psychotropic drugs), but they block the re-uptake of noradrenaline by adrenergic nerve terminals. They have pronounced anticholinergic action causing blurred vision, dry mouth, constipation and urinary retention. The other side-effects include orthostatic hypotension, precipitation of cardiac failure and tachycardia.

82 A False
   B False
   C True
   D False
   E True

Codeine is methylmorphine and heroin is derived following the acetylation of both phenolic and alcoholic hydroxyl groups of morphine. Papaverine, a major opium alkaloid of benzoisoquinoline group lacks morphine-like effects and is a smooth muscle relaxant. As compared with morphine, codeine and thebaine belong to the phenanthrene class and noscapine and papaverine belong to the benzylisoquinoline group.

83 Halothane
A   0.01% thymol is used to enhance stability
B   Causes vasoconstriction in the skeletal muscle
C   Pre-treatment with phenobarbitone increases the sensitivity of liver to repeated exposure
D   Ostwald partition coefficient is 93
E   Has no effect on cardiac contractility

84 Nitrous oxide
A   Has a blood/gas partition coefficient of 0.47 at 37°C
B   Is carried in a physical solution
C   At 10% nitrous oxide, maximal degree of analgesia can be obtained
D   30% nitrous oxide elevates the resting respiratory minute volume
E   Has a low anaesthetic potency

85 Atropine
A   Causes a decrease in physiological dead space
B   Reduces the voltage and frequency of alpha rhythm in the EEG
C   Can paralyse accommodation of the eye
D   Increases the intrabiliary pressure
E   In large doses causes a rise in the basal alveolar ventilation

86 Indomethacin
A   Modifies the effect of oral anticoagulants
B   Is useful in psoriatic arthritis
C   Rectal suppositories provide a consistent therapeutic effect
D   20% of the drug is excreted unchanged in the urine
E   Inhibits the biosynthesis of prostaglandins

83 A True
B False
C True
D False
E False

Halothane causes vasodilatation in the skeletal muscle and decreases the cardiac contractility. It has a rubber solubility coefficient (also called Ostwald partition coefficient) of 121.

84 A True
B True
C False
D False
E True

Nitrous oxide at 20% is as effective as 15 mg of morphine sulphate and at 35% it gives a maximal degree of analgesia. 50% nitrous oxide elevates the resting minute volume and not 30%.

85 A False
B True
C True
D False
E True

Atropine causes bronchodilatation and a rise in respiratory rate thus increasing the physiological dead space. It has mild antispasmodic action on the gallbladder and bile ducts.

86 A False
B True
C False
D True
E True

Indomethacin is an indoleacetic acid derivative. Its main actions are analgesic, anti-inflammatory and anti-pyretic. It acts by inhibiting prostaglandin synthesis by causing reversible blockade of the conversion of arachidonic acid to PGG_2. Indomethacin causes hypertension, salt and water retention, reversible abnormalities of liver function tests. It inhibits platelet aggregation and prolongs the bleeding time (which still remains within the normal range). It is well absorbed after oral/rectal administration and the bioavailability is 80%. It is metabolized in the liver.

87 Tricyclic antidepressants
  A Elevate mood in healthy persons
  B Take 2–3 weeks to act
  C Have no cardiac effects
  D Directly stimulate adrenergic receptors
  E Have weak anticholinergic effects

88 Fentanyl
  A Is related to phenylpiperidines
  B Low doses produce muscular rigidity
  C Is ten times more potent than morphine
  D A combination with droperidol is called Innovar
  E Can be reversed with naloxone

87 A False
B True
C False
D False
E False

Tricyclic antidepressants facilitate noradrenergic and serotonergic neurotransmission by inhibiting re-uptake of the released neurotransmitter into the presynaptic nerve ending. The clinical response to tricyclics usually occurs after a delay of several weeks. Tricyclics are indicated in the treatment of endogenous depression. The side-effects following the use of tricyclics are confusion, tremors (cholinergic effect), orthostatic hypotension, cardiac arrhythmias, agranulocytosis and hepatotoxicity.

88 A True
B False
C False
D True
E True

Fentanyl is a synthetic opioid related to phenylpiperidines. It is a central nervous system depressant producing marked analgesia, respiratory depression. Plasma fentanyl concentrations of 4–10 ng/ml are adequate for analgesia if combined with nitrous oxide during surgery. Following IV administration, it causes delayed respiratory depression due to secondary rise in plasma fentanyl concentration. Fentanyl in high doses causes chest wall rigidity making ventilation difficult. High-dose fentanyl anaesthesia has been shown to modify or abolish the 'stress' response to anaesthesia. Fentanyl is highly lipid soluble and is rapidly and extensively distributed to tissues.

89 Sevoflurane
A   Is a halogenated ether
B   Has a blood/gas partition coefficient of 0.3
C   Has a MAC value between 1.7 and 2.3%
D   Causes dose-related cardiovascular depression more marked than halothane
E   Does not react with soda lime

90 Desflurane
A   Is a halogenated ether
B   Has a boiling point of 32°C
C   Has a MAC value around 5.4%
D   Has a blood/gas partition coefficient of 0.4
E   Causes sinus bradycardia during induction

89 A True
B False
C True
D False
E False

Sevoflurane is a halogenated methyl isopropyl ether which was first synthesized in the early 1970s and is currently used in Japan. It is potent, non-explosive and non-inflammable in clinical concentration. It reacts with soda lime to form traces of related ether which have not, so far, been shown to cause toxic effects in animals exposed chronically in a closed system. Induction of anaesthesia by Sevoflurane is rapid and smooth. It has a blood/gas partition coefficient of 0.6 with MAC values between 1.7 and 2.3%. Sevoflurane causes dos-related cardiovascular and respiratory depression. Depression of cardiac output is less marked than that produced by halothane, but more than that caused by isoflurane. It potentiates the effects of calcium channel-blocking agents and sensitizes the heart to circulating catecholamines to an extent intermediate between that of enflurane and isoflurane. Sevoflurane has similar effects to that of isoflurane on cerebral circulation.

90 A True
B False
C True
D False
E False

Desflurane (I-653) is a fluorinated methyl ether structurally related to isoflurane. It is non-flammable and non-explosive and is stable in the presence of soda lime. It has a boiling point of 23°C, hence it needs to be used with a special vaporizer within a closed circle system. The MAC value for humans has been found to be around 5.4%. Desflurane has a blood/gas partition coefficient of 0.4, with a pleasant odour. It produces smooth, rapid gaseous induction of anaesthesia. Recovery from anaesthesia is faster regardless of the duration of anasthesia or the inspired concentration of anaesthetic used. In humans it causes sinus tachycardia during induction of anaesthesia, caused possibly by excitement.

91 Sufentanil
- A Is ten times more potent than fentanyl
- B Unlike fentanyl it does not cause muscle rigidity
- C Causes histamine release
- D Is bound to plasma proteins
- E Can cause hypotension

92 Opiate antagonists
- A Nalorphine causes marked dysphoria and hallucinations
- B Naloxone has the highest affinity for Kappa receptor
- C Naloxone precipitates withdrawal syndrome
- D A single IV dose of 0.4 mg naloxone lasts for 5 min
- E Naltrexone is a short-acting opiate antagonist

93 Pipecuronium
- A Is an analogue of pancuronium
- B Causes release of histamine
- C Has similar onset of action as pancuronium
- D Is bound to plasma proteins
- E Is excreted via the bile

91 A True
    B False
    C False
    D True
    E True
Sufentanil is 5 to 10 times more potent than fentanyl. It causes predictable side-effects such as respiratory depression, bradycardia, nausea, vomiting, smooth muscle spasm and muscle rigidity. Like fentanyl, sufentanil does not cause histamine release. Sufentanil is bound to plasma proteins (92.5%), the principal binding protein being α_1-acid glycoprotein. Sufentanil, when used as a sole IV induction agent, causes hypotension.

92 A True
    B False
    C True
    D False
    E False
Nalorphine is closely related to morphine and has similar but weaker effects. Naloxone is a competitive antagonist of Mu, Kappa, Sigma, Delta opioid receptors, but has been shown to have the highest affinity for the Mu receptor. A single IV dose of naloxone 0.4 mg antagonizes the effects of morphine for 30–45 minutes. Naltrexone is a long-acting opiate antagonist and is used in the treatment of narcotic addiction.

93 A True
    B False
    C True
    D True
    E False
It has no cardiovascular effects. Its neuromuscular blocking properties are similar to, or slightly greater than, that of pancuronium. Pipecuronium has a faster clearance and larger volume of distribution than pancuronium. The kidney seems to be an important route of elimination.

94 Doxacurium
A Is a short-acting muscle relaxant
B Is a monoquaternary diester
C Is broken down by Hofmann elimination
D Is cardiovascularly stable
E Can be given in doses of 0.02–0.03 mg/kg

95 Mivacurium
A Is a diester compound
B Is a depolarizing neuromuscular blocker
C Is ideal for short surgical procedures
D Causes release of histamine
E Can cause hypotension

96 Cerebrospinal fluid (CSF)
A Its composition depends on active transport
B Composition is similar to brain intracellular fluid
C Rate of production is 300–400 ml/24 h
D CSF chloride levels are high
E CSF glucose parallels the plasma glucose levels

94 A False
B False
C False
D True
E False
Doxacurium is a long-acting, non-depolarizing muscle relaxant with a duration of action similar to that of pancuronium. It is a bisquaternary benzylisoquinolinium diester with chemical structure similar to atracurium. It is not broken down by Hofmann degradation.

95 A True
B False
C True
D True
E True
Mivacurium is a non-depolarizing neuromuscular blocker with a short duration of action. It is a bisbenzylisoquinolinium diester compound. It is rapidly hydrolysed by plasma cholinesterase. The rapid rate of hydrolysis indicates that mivacurium has a short elimination half-life and thus can be an ideal agent for short surgical procedures. Mivacurium in small doses produces minimal cardiovascular effects, but doses above 0.15 mg/kg (twice the ED_{95}) cause hypotension. A transient fall in blood pressure has been described, which is probably due to histamine release.

96 A True
B False
C False
D True
E False
The composition of cerebrospinal fluid (CSF) is similar to the brain extracellular fluid. Its rate of production is 100–250 ml/24 h and normal total volume is 100–200 ml. CSF glucose is 60% of its concentration in plasma because of the incomplete penetration of blood/brain barrier.

97 Sleep
A   Dream recall is characteristic of 80% of awakening from rapid eye movement sleep (REM sleep)
B   During REM sleep body temperature falls
C   First period of REM sleep occurs 90 min after sleep begins
D   In stage 2 of non-REM sleep, EEG comprises 12–16 Hz spindles
E   In paradoxical sleep the muscle tone is increased

98 Endorphins
A   Are released during acupuncture
B   Naloxone reverses the analgesia caused by halothane
C   The amount of endorphins released is directly proportional to the degree and duration of exercise period
D   Injection into the lateral ventricles of the brain produces bradycardia and hypotension
E   In neurogenic shock, naloxone improves blood pressure and heart rate

99 Spinal cord transection
A   Spinal shock lasts in human beings for 6 weeks
B   Patients breakdown large amounts of proteins
C   Leads to hypocalcaemia
D   Mass reflex gives a degree of bladder and bowel control
E   Blood pressure remains stable

100 Hypothalamus
A   Supraoptic nuclei are responsible for the release of oxytocin and vasopressin
B   Posterior hypothalamus controls response to heat
C   Limbic system and hypothalamus control fear and rage
D   Lateral superior hypothalamus regulates thirst
E   Anterior hypothalamus regulates the secretion of ACTH

97 A True
  B False
  C True
  D True
  E False
Non-REM sleep consists of four stages: Stage 1 – low amplitude; Stage 3 – 20%–50% high-amplitude slow waves; Stage 4 – slow waves.

98 A True
  B True
  C True
  D False
  E True
Naloxone 10 mg/kg IV increases up to 70% of rats responding to painful stimulation during halothane anaesthesia suggesting that endorphins are released by volatile anaesthetics. Injection of endorphins into the lateral ventricles causes tachycardia and hypertension, whereas injection into cisterna magna produces bradycardia and hypotension. Naloxone is shown to increase dopamine levels in shock and improve cardiovascular function.

99 A False
  B True
  C False
  D True
  E False
Spinal shock in humans lasts for 2 weeks and hypercalcaemia is seen quite frequently. The blood pressure fluctuates considerably due to the loss of baroreceptor reflexes.

100 A True
  B False
  C True
  D True
  E False
The anterior hypothalamus controls the response to heat and the ventral hypothalamus regulates the secretion of ACTH.

101 Dynorphin
A   Is a weak opioid peptide
B   Causes analgesia in small doses
C   Produces a wide range of motor and behavioural effects
D   Electroencephalogram shows large amplitude, slow wave activity after injection of dynorphin in the periaqueductal grey matter
E   Animals treated with dynorphin develop 'opisthotonic posture'

102 Muscle spindle
A   Consists of 20 muscle fibres enclosed in the intrafusal fibres
B   Secondary or flower-spray endings are located at the ends of the intrafusal fibres
C   Motor nerve supply consists of A delta fibres
D   Extrafusal fibres are non-contractile elements
E   Intrafusal fibres lie parallel to the rest of muscle fibres

103 Cerebral circulation
A   Cerebral metabolic rate for oxygen ($CMRO_2$) is about 2 ml/100 g brain per min
B   Hypercapnia causes cerebral vasodilatation
C   A low PO_2 is associated with severe vasoconstriction
D   When intracranial pressure is raised to 33 mmHg, cerebral blood flow is increased
E   Glucose is the major source of energy for the brain

104 Nerve fibres
A   A delta fibres have a conduction velocity of 5–10 metres per second
B   C unmyelinated fibres carry pain and reflex response fibres
C   A alpha fibres have an absolute refractory period of 1.2 ms
D   Local anaesthetics affect touch fibres in the A group followed by depressing group C fibres
E   B type of fibres are susceptible to hypoxia

101 A False
  B False
  C True
  D True
  E False
Dynorphin is an extremely potent opioid peptide which produces analgesia in large doses. When injected in the periaqueductal grey matter it causes motor and behavioural and EEG changes. Animals treated with dynorphin develop 'catatonic posture'.

102 A False
  B True
  C True
  D False
  E True
Muscle spindle consists of two to ten enclosed intrafusal fibres and the extrafusal fibres are contractile elements. As the A delta fibres are very small they are also known as small motor neurone system or gamma efferents of Leksell.

103 A False
  B True
  C False
  D False
  E True
Cerebral metabolic rate for oxygen ($CMRO_2$) is 3.5 ml/100 g of brain per min or 49 ml/min for the whole brain in an adult. Hypercapnia and hypoxia cause vasodilatation. When the intracranial pressure is increased to 33 mmHg the cerebral blood flow is actually decreased for a few minutes.

104 A False
  B True
  C False
  D False
  E True
A delta fibres have a conduction velocity of 12–30 metres per second and they carry pain, touch and temperature fibres. All the A fibres have an absolute refractory period of 0.4–1 ms. The local anaesthetics depress the group C fibres first, followed by the touch fibres in group A.

105 Sensory system and endogenous opiate receptors
  A   Supraspinal structures (periaqueductal grey matter) contain delta receptors
  B   Opiate receptors are situated alongside chemoreceptor trigger zone
  C   Lateral thalamus deals with highly localized somatic pain
  D   Opioid peptides facilitate the release of substance P
  E   Opiate receptors are localized in the marginal cell zone

106 Synaptic transmission
  A   The fast potential change which appears just before the action potential is called excitatory post-synaptic potential (EPSP)
  B   EPSP is monophasic and non-propagating
  C   Depolarization following an inhibitory stimulus is called inhibitory post-synaptic potential (IPSP)
  D   IPSP results from an increased flow of potassium and chloride making the inside of the membrane more negative
  E   EPSP arises due to efflux of chloride ions through the post-synaptic membrane

107 Substantia gelatinosa and pain pathways
  A   Marginal layer sends impulses via ipsilateral anterolateral funiculus
  B   Small fibres from layers VII and VIII make up the intermediate grey matter
  C   Spinoreticular fibres terminate in reticular formation
  D   Lamina I, IV and V send input via spinothalamic projection
  E   Periaqueductal grey matter contains endorphins

105 A False
B True
C True
D False
E True
Supraspinal structures (PAG), along with medial thalamic nuclei,
contain Mu receptors. Substantia gelatinosa contains both Mu
and Delta receptors. Medial thalamic nuclei mediate poorly
localized and emotionally influenced pain. Opioid peptides inhibit
the release of substance P. The opiate receptors are also located
in the dorsal layer of substantia gelatinosa corresponding to
Lamina I and II of Rexed.

106 A False
B True
C False
D True
E False
A slow potential change which appears before the action potential
is called excitatory post-synaptic potential (EPSP). These EPSPs
are due to an influx of ions like sodium, potassium and chloride.
Hyperpolarization following an inhibitory stimulus is called
inhibitory post-synaptic potential.

107 A False
B False
C True
D True
E False
Marginal layer sends impulses via contralateral anterolateral
funiculus. Large fibres from layers VII and VIII make up the
intermediate grey matter. Periaqueductal grey matter contains
enkephalins.

108 Electroencephalogram and sleep
  A Alpha rhythm is seen when the subject is awake but relaxed with eyes open
  B When a subject is asleep, larger slower delta waves are seen
  C Dreaming occurs during REM sleep
  D Pontine sleep centre is responsible for slow wave sleep
  E REM sleep constitutes 40% of total time spent asleep

109 Cerebrospinal fluid (CSF)
  A Sodium content is 152 mmol
  B Is isotonic with plasma
  C Glucose content of CSF is two-thirds of arterial blood
  D Protein content is 600 mg/100 ml
  E Choroid plexus forms approximately 1000 ml of CSF/day

110 Action potential
  A Occurs due to different ionic concentration of sodium and potassium
  B The negative potential inside the nerve fibre pulls positively charged potassium ions to the outside
  C When sodium ions enter inside the membrane, depolarization occurs
  D In a resting state the potential recorded inside the nerve fibre is $+85\,mV$
  E At the peak of the action potential, the voltage changes to $+35\,V$

111 Endogenous opiates
  A Endorphins are derived from proenkephalin B
  B Prodynorphins are precursors of dynorphin
  C In 1975 highly specific opiate receptors were identified
  D Enkephalins were discovered in 1973
  E Proenkephalins and prodynorphins have molecular weight between 28 000 and 32 000

108 A False
    B True
    C True
    D False
    E False

Alpha rhythm is seen when the subject is awake but relaxed with *eyes closed*. Pontine sleep centre is responsible for the generation of paradoxical sleep. REM sleep constitutes 20% of the total time spent asleep.

109 A False
    B True
    C True
    D False
    E False

The sodium content of CSF is 147 mmol and the protein content is 20 mg/100 ml.

110 A True
    B False
    C True
    D False
    E False

The negative potential inside the nerve fibre pulls positively charged potassium ions to the inside. In a resting state the potential recorded inside the nerve fibre is -85 mV. At the peak of the action potential, the voltage changes to $+35$ mV.

111 A False
    B True
    C False
    D False
    E True

Endorphins are derived from pro-opiomelanocortin. In 1973 highly specific opiate receptors were identified in the CNS of vertebrates. Enkephalins were discovered in 1975.

112 Endorphins
A   Are located in the gastric antrum and pancreas
B   In the hypothalamus they are synthesized in the arcuate nucleus
C   Are present in high concentrations in the placenta
D   Have a short half-life as compared with enkephalins
E   Cause profound analgesia

113 Neurotransmitters
A   Serotonin is secreted by the limbic system
B   Noradrenaline is secreted by the cerebellum
C   Substance P is released by the small intestine
D   Post-ganglionic parasympathetic endings secrete acetylcholine
E   γ-aminobutyric acid (GABA) is secreted by the retina

114 Gate control theory of pain
A   Depends on afferent inhibition for function
B   Depends on an overstimulation of small fibres for opening the gate
C   Has been proved to act in the spinal cord
D   Would predict that stimulation of somatosensory endings in the skin over an area of pain might relieve painful stimulation
E   Involves corticofugal signals that have no effect upon pain sensitivity

115 Enkephalins
A   Depend on calcium ions for their release
B   Highest concentrations are present in the medulla
C   Molecular weight is 30 000
D   Have a half-life of 1 min
E   Are released simultaneously with catecholamines

112 A True
B True
C True
D False
E True
Endorphins are synthesized in the arcuate nucleus of the hypothalamus and also in the median eminence close to the ventromedial border of the third ventricle. They are present in high concentration in the gastric antrum, pancreas, placenta in pregnant women and neonates. Endorphins have a long half-life of 1 h as compared with enkephalins.

113 A True
B True
C True
D True
E True
Noradrenaline is secreted by cerebellum, cerebral cortex, hypothalamus, brain stem and spinal cord.

114 A False
B False
C False
D True
E False
The term 'gate control' is applied to rapidly acting mechanisms which accept and control the passage of impulses from the afferent fibre input to cells which may then trigger the various effector systems and evoke sensation.

115 A True
B False
C False
D True
E True
Enkephalins are present in the globus pallidus, perioptic area of the hypothalamus, limbic system, posterior lobe of pituitary and the dorsal horn of the spinal cord. The molecular weight of enkephalins ranges from 500 to 20 000. Enkephalins are found in the sympathetic ganglion and adrenal medulla, hence are released simultaneously with catecholamines.

116 When skeletal muscle shortens in response to stimulation
A There is a decrease in the width of I band
B There is a decrease in the width of A band
C There is a decrease in the width of A *and* I bands
D An increase in the width of H zone
E All the above can occur

117 A reflex
A Requires an intact cerebral cortex
B Uses a multisynaptic pathway
C Is destroyed several weeks after spinal transection
D Is a stereotyped response to a stimulus
E Is not neural in nature

118 Hypothalamus
A Stimulation of superior hypothalamus causes contraction of urinary bladder
B Stimulation of lateral hypothalamus causes a fall in blood pressure
C Stimulation of posterior hypothalamus produces increased secretion of adrenaline and noradrenaline
D Stimulation of posterior hypothalamus causes prolonged sleep
E 'Satiety centre' is located in the ventromedial nucleus

116 A True
   B False
   C False
   D False
   E False
There is no change in the width of A band during shortening of the skeletal muscle.

117 A False
   B False
   C False
   D True
   E False
Reflex arc is a basic unit of neural activity and it consists of a sense organ, an afferent neurone, synapse, an efferent neurone and an effector. The afferent neurones enter the dorsal root (sensory) and the efferent neurones leave via the ventral root (motor). This relationship between sensory and motor neurones is known as the Bell–Magendie Law.
The simplest reflex arc is one with a single synapse between the afferent and efferent neurones (monosynaptic reflex); reflex arcs with more than one interneurone is called polysynaptic. When a skeletal muscle is stretched it contracts; this response is called the stretch reflex. The stimulus that starts the reflex is stretch of the muscle and the response is contraction of the muscle which is being stretched. The sense organ is called the muscle spindle.

118 A False
   B False
   C True
   D False
   E True
Stimulation of superior anterior hypothalamus causes contraction of the urinary bladder, a parasympathetic response. Stimulation of lateral hypothalamus produces a rise in blood pressure, pupillary dilatation, piloerection, signs of diffuse adrenergic discharge. Destruction and not stimulation of posterior hypothalamus causes prolonged sleep. Stimulation of 'satiety centre' causes cessation of eating, whereas the lesions in this region cause hyperphagia and, if the food supply is abundant, leads to hypothalamic obesity.

119 Reflexes
A Cerebal cortex is involved in optical righting reflexes
B Tonic labyrinthine reflexes are integrated in spinal cord
C Muscle spindles are involved in stretch reflex
D Midbrain integrates the contraction of muscles
E Stretch is a stimulus for negative supporting reflex

120 Posture and movement
A Stimulation of Broadmann's area 6 produces rotation of the eyes to opposite side
B Pyramidal system controls unskilled, fine movement
C Babinski sign consists of dorsiflexion of great toe and fanning of other toes
D Destruction of pyramidal system has no effect
E Fine movements commands arise in the association areas of the cortex

121 Basal ganglia
A Chorea is associated with degeneration of putamen
B Athetosis is associated with intermittent, slow, writhing movements
C In Wilson's disease the ceruloplasmin levels are high
D In Ballism, subthalamic nuclei are damaged
E Both hyperkinetic and hypokinetic features are seen in Parkinson's disease

119 A   True
    B   False
    C   True
    D   False
    E   True
The stimulus for optical righting reflexes comes from visual receptors, i.e. eyes and the response consists of righting of head. Tonic labyrinthine reflexes are integrated in midbrain following the receipt of stimulus from gravity via otolith organs, the response being extensor rigidity. Spinal cord and medulla oblongata integrate stretch reflexes causing contraction of muscle. Stretch stimulus is propagated via proprioceptors in extensors and integrated in the spinal cord causing release of positive supporting action.

120 A   True
    B   False
    C   True
    D   False
    E   True
Brodmann's area 6, also called premotor cortex or premotor area, when stimulated causes adverse movements such as gross rotation of the eyes, head and trunk to the opposite side. Pyramidal system controls skilled, fine movements and its destruction causes weakness and clumsiness.

121 A   False
    B   False
    C   False
    D   True
    E   True
Chorea is due to the degeneration of caudate nucleus and is characterized by rapid, involuntary 'dancing movements'. Athetosis is due to lesion of the lenticular nucleus and is associated with continuous, slow writhing movements. Wilson's disease is a familial disorder of copper metabolism in which the plasma copper-binding protein ceruloplasmin is usually low. Hyperkinetic features in Parkinson's disease include rigidity and tremors and the hypokinetic features, akinesia or poverty of movements.

122 Temperature control

A   Brain and arterial blood are the two sites where temperature is strictly maintained

B   A rise in core temperature to 40°C causes apathy and impairment of ability to make judgement

C   Enzymatic activity is effective at 37°C

D   Temperature control centre lies in the medulla oblongata

E   Hyperventilation is a chief mechanism of body temperature loss in dogs

123 γ-aminobutyric acid (GABA)

A   Mediates presynaptic inhibition in the spinal cord

B   Its action is facilitated by picrotoxin

C   Is decreased in slow wave sleep

D   Is formed by hydroxylation of glutamic acid

E   Pyridoxal phosphate is a cofactor in GABA formation

122 A True
      B False
      C True
      D False
      E True

In the periphery lie the cold and warm receptors which carry the information to the hypothalamus and other integrating areas, which respond with appropriate efferent output. Thus firing of cold receptors stimulates heat-producing and heat-conserving mechanisms. Body temperature is regulated by altering heat production or heat loss. Heat production is increased by increasing muscle tone, shivering and voluntary activity. Heat loss occurs by conduction, convection and radiation and evaporation of water from body surface.

123 A True
      B False
      C False
      D False
      E True

γ-Aminobutyric acid (GABA), a neuroinhibitory transmitter, is released in large amounts from the brain during slow wave sleep. Its action is antagonized by picrotoxin. GABA is formed by decarboxylation of glutamic acid and it requires pyridoxine phosphate (a derivative of vitamin B complex) as a cofactor. Deficiency of pyridoxine leads to signs of neural hyperexcitability and convulsions.

2   Cardiovascular system

1   Propranolol
A   Causes peripheral vasodilatation
B   Has no effect on growth hormone
C   Inhibits gluconeogenesis
D   Plasma half-life is 6 h
E   Causes a rise in airway resistance

2   Physiological solutions
A   0.9% sodium chloride contains 154 meq of sodium/l
B   3% solution of sodium chloride contains 855 meq of sodium and chloride/l
C   Hypertonic sodium chloride can precipitate pulmonary oedema
D   Ringer's solution contains 2 meq of calcium/l
E   Ammonium chloride can precipitate hepatic coma

3   Sodium nitroprusside (SNP)
A   Is a direct smooth muscle relaxant
B   Arterial blood pressure returns to prehypotensive levels within 3 min of stopping SNP infusion
C   The rhodanase enzyme catalyses conjugation of cyanide
D   Vitamin B12 can be used to treat SNP overdose
E   Initial treatment of choice in overdose is cobalt edetate

Cardiovascular system: Answers

1　A　True
　　B　True
　　C　False
　　D　False
　　E　True
Propranolol is an aromatic amine. It has both negative inotropic and chronotropic effect. It has no intrinsic sympathomimeticraction but acts by competitive antagonism of $\beta1$ and $\beta2$ adrenoreceptors. It decreases myocardial oxygen consumption and increases the peripheral vascular resistance. Propranolol causes a fall in FEV_1 by increasing airway resistance. It causes hypoglycaemia due to blockade of gluconeogenesis. It decreases plasma renin activity and suppresses aldosterone release. The elimination half-life of propranolol is 2–4 hours and it is excreted via urine.

2　A　True
　　B　False
　　C　True
　　D　False
　　E　True
3% Sodium chloride solution contains 513 mEq each of sodium and chloride/l. Ringer's solution contains 4 mEq of calcium and potassium/l each with 147 mEq of sodium/l. Ammonium chloride is used to treat metabolic alkalosis due to vomiting and loss of hydrochloric acid.

3　A　True
　　B　False
　　C　True
　　D　True
　　E　False
Sodium nitroprusside (SNP) acts through an intermediate vasodilator site which involves sulphydryl group bound to smooth muscle membrane. Arterial pressure returns to pre-hypotensive levels within 6 min provided blood loss, if any, is corrected.

4 Nifedipine
- A After oral administration 70% of the drug is absorbed
- B Can be given intravenously
- C Plasma half-life is 4–5 h
- D Is metabolized in the liver
- E Is useful in Prinzmetal angina

5 β-blocking drugs
- A Metoprolol has a membrane-stabilizing effect
- B Act by altering the neural function
- C Patients with asthma are sensitive to cardioselective beta blockers
- D Antihypertensive action of propranolol is proportional to the pretreatment renin levels
- E Timolol is a cardioselective drug

6 Reserpine
- A Is derived from Rauwolfia serpentina
- B Causes postural hypotension in usual oral doses
- C Increases gastric acid secretion
- D Can make a patient a 'suicidal risk'
- E Can potentiate hypotension during anaesthesia

4 A False
  B True
  C True
  D True
  E True
About 90% of the drug nifedipine is absorbed after oral administration. About 75% of the metabolites are excreted via the kidneys and 15% by the gastrointestinal tract. In Prinzmetal angina it dilates coronary vessels without decreasing myocardial contractility.

5 A False
  B False
  C True
  D True
  F False
Propranolol is a membrane-stabilizing agent which can precipitate bronchospasm. β-blockers act on the post-synaptic neurones, i.e. the effector tissue. Propranolol is most active in lowering blood pressure when pretreatment levels are high and the hypotensive effect is correlated with the ability of the drug to inhibit renin release. Timolol is a non-selective blocker which is used in the treatment of glaucoma.

6 A True
  B False
  C True
  D True
  E True
Reserpine acts by depleting neurones of noradrenaline and thus reducing sympathetic nervous system tone. It is a major active ingredient of the plant *Rauwolfia serpentina*. In the brain reserpine depletes levels of 5-hydroxytryptamine, dopamine, histamine, adrenaline and noradrenaline. It causes sedation due to depletion of dopamine. At the periphery, reserpine reduces sympathetic tone by depleting noradrenaline stores in the postsynaptic neurone. Reserpine causes a fall in peripheral resistance, cardiac output and blood pressure due to loss of sympathetic tone.

7 **Antidysrhythmics**
   A β-blockers slow the rate of rise in Phase 4 and Phase 0
   B Quinidine and procainamide slow the rate of rise in Phase 4
   C Amiodarone prolongs the refractory period
   D Verapamil acts as a calcium agonist
   E Quinidine is used in the treatment of extrasystoles

8 **Sympathomimetics**
   A Noradrenaline has no action on the cardiac output
   B Methoxamine acts mainly on the Alpha receptors
   C Mephentermine has a direct mode of action
   D Salbutamol has a significant effect on the peripheral resistance
   E Methylamphetamine can increase the renal blood flow

9 **Hydralazine**
   A Is a monoamine oxidase (MAO) inhibitor
   B Causes reflex-induced bradycardia
   C Parenteral dose is 10–40 mg repeated 12 hourly
   D Causes an increase in renal blood flow
   E Is a hydrazine derivative

7 A False
  B True
  C True
  D False
  E True
A number of antidysrhythmic agents block myocardial Na^+ or Ca^{2+} channels in a state-dependent manner, i.e. they bind with a higher affinity to activated or inactivated channels than to resting channels. The agents that depress myocardial Na^+ channels and thus reduce V_{max} are placed in class I, those that have sympathetic blocking actions go in class II, agents that prolong action potential duration and refractoriness go in class III and agents with Ca^{2+} channel-blocking properties in class IV.

8 A True
  B True
  C False
  D False
  E True
Sympathomimetics are classified into direct-acting and indirect acting. A number of directly acting sympathomimetics differ from adrenaline in that they are more selective in activating α- and β-receptors. Phenylephrine and methoxamine are synthetic selective α-receptor agonists. Dobutamine and dopamine are specific for β1-receptors.

9 A True
  B False
  C True
  D True
  E True
Hydralazine, although it is a MAO inhibitor, is of no clinical use. It causes a reflex-induced tachycardia. The parenteral dose is 10–40 mg IM repeated every 4–6 hours.

10 Nitroglycerin
A Causes 'post arteriolar dilatation'
B Hypotension is potentiated if the patient is supine and immobile
C Can be applied topically
D When absorbed the peak effect occurs in 2 min
E Prolonged use can lead to tolerance

11 Noradrenaline
A Causes vasoconstriction of blood vessels in muscles
B Increases the heart rate by reflex action
C Has no action on the force of cardiac contraction
D Can cause anxiety on IV injection
E Causes dry mouth

12 Calcium antagonists
A Verapamil decreases the MAC of halothane by 10%
B Nifedipine increases the potency of muscle relaxants
C Can interfere with glucose tolerance
D Verapamil can be used for inducing hypotensive anaesthesia
E Can be used in prophylaxis of malignant hyperpyrexia

13 β-blockers
A Oxprenolol has a similar action to propranolol on cardiac and extracardiac sites
B Propranolol exerts a sedative effect
C Practolol has a membrane-stabilizing effect
D Dysrhythmias due to digitalis overdose respond well to β-blockers
E Propranolol is effective in Fallot's tetralogy

10 A True
    B False
    C True
    D False
    E True
Nitroglycerin causes both post arteriolar and venous dilatation and the hypotension caused by it is potentiated in subjects who are upright and mobile. It is equally effective sublingually or topically and when absorbed the peak effect occurs in 30 s.

11 A True
    B False
    C False
    D False
    E True
Noradrenaline increases the heart rate by direct action on the heart. Unlike adrenaline it is much less active and does not cause anxiety. It causes dry mouth due to vasoconstriction and decreased secretion.

12 A False
    B True
    C True
    D True
    E True
Verapamil (0.5 mg/kg) decreases the MAC of halothane by 25%. The secretion of insulin is influenced by the influx of calcium and thus calcium antagonists affect glucose tolerance.

13 A False
    B True
    C False
    D False
    E True
Oxprenolol has a similar action to propranolol on cardiac sites only. Propranolol has a membrane-stabilizing effect and drugs such as phenytoin are effective in controlling the dysrhythmias caused by digitalis overdose.

14 Digoxin
  A   Is derived from digitalis purpurea and used as the most
       common therapeutic glycoside
  B   Digitalis was used for dropsy in the 17th century
  C   Digitalis glycosides are related to sex hormones
  D   The aglycone portion is a sugar which makes glycoside soluble
  E   Neurological complications are the last to occur in digitalis
       intoxication

15 Disopyramide
  A   Has no ill effects in the presence of cardiac failure
  B   Can precipitate glaucoma
  C   Slows conduction in the His-Purkinje fibres
  D   Dose is 2 mg/kg IV
  E   Is not effective in controlling arrhythmias following myocardial
       infarction

16 Ephedrine
  A   Has a direct action on alpha and beta receptors
  B   Enhances spinal reflexes
  C   Increases the renal blood flow
  D   Is broken down and excreted in the urine
  E   The treatment of its overdose consists of barbiturates

14 A False
    B True
    C True
    D False
    E False
Digoxin is derived from *D. lanata*. The glycone (and not aglycone) portion makes glycoside soluble and neurological complications, such as tinnitus, headache, blurred vision, are the first signs of digitalis toxicity.

15 A False
    B True
    C True
    D True
    E False
Disopyramide is a tertiary amine and is used in the treatment of atrial or ventricular dysrhythmias including Wolff–Parkinson–White syndrome. It is a class Ia antiarrhythmic agent and acts by blocking the fast inward sodium current leading to the prolongation of duration of action potential and effective refractory period. Disopyramide slows conduction through the His-Purkinje system and acts as a negative inotrope. It causes anticholinergic side-effects. The IV loading dose is 2 mg/kg and the adult oral dose is 300–800 mg/day in divided doses.

16 A True
    B True
    C False
    D False
    E True
Ephedrine does not have any action on the renal blood flow and is excreted unbroken in the urine.

17 Labetalol
 A Is effective in hypertension following infarction
 B Can be used in association with cimetidine
 C Has a diuretic effect
 D Dosage should be decreased in liver disease
 E Causes postural hypotension

18 Trimetaphan
 A Is broken down by enzymatic hydrolysis
 B Causes a fall in blood pressure associated with bradycardia
 C Is used to improve perfusion following cardiac surgery
 D Is compatible with thiopentone
 E Tachyphylaxis occurs following continuous administration

19 Dopamine
 A Increases the myocardial oxygen consumption
 B Causes a decrease in the peripheral blood flow
 C Has a significant effect on the diastolic blood pressure
 D Increases the sodium excretion
 E Rates greater than 50 mcg/kg per min have been used safely in
    advanced circulatory decompensation

17 A True
  B False
  C False
  D True
  E True

Labetalol is effective in controlling hypertension following myocardial infarction at the rate of 15 mg/h increasing gradually to 120 mg/h. Cimetidine interacts with it, thus increasing the plasma concentration of labetalol. Labetalol causes difficulty in micturition.

18 A True
  B False
  C True
  D False
  E True

Trimetaphan, a ganglion blocker, causes hypotension associated with tachycardia. It is broken down partly by enzymatic hydrolysis and partly excreted unchanged in the urine.

19 A False
  B True
  C False
  D True
  E True

Dopamine is a naturally occurring catecholamine. It is used in the management of low cardiac output states, septic shock and in the prevention of renal failure. In low dose (2 mcg/kg per min) it acts upon specific dopaminergic receptors and in high doses (5–10 mcg/kg per min) it stimulates the beta cells. At low doses it causes positive inotropism, increase in cardiac output and coronary blood flow. At high doses of above 15 mcg/kg per min it causes peripheral vasoconstriction by α-adrenergic effect. In low doses (1–5 mcg/kg per min) dopamine causes an increase in renal blood flow by decreasing the renal vascular resistance.

20 Captopril
    A Is used in the control of mild hypertension
    B Causes increased bronchial secretions
    C Side-effects include hyperkalaemia and neutrophilia
    D Rarely leads to Stevens–Johnson syndrome
    E Is an anti-dysrhythmic

21 Adrenaline
    A Increases the movements of the stomach and intestine
    B Can decrease the body's total oxygen consumption by 30%
    C Dilates coronary vessels
    D Its action can be antagonized by tolazoline
    E Causes a rise in blood sugar by releasing ACTH

22 Retroperitoneal fibrosis occurs following treatment with:
    A Propranolol
    B Methysergide
    C Tyramine
    D Progesterone
    E Clonidine

23 Procainamide
    A Is effective following myocardial infarction
    B Is contraindicated in heart failure
    C Causes granulocytosis
    D Dose is reduced in patients with renal insufficiency
    E Maximum IV dose is 2 g

20 A True
   B False
   C False
   D True
   E False
Captopril is used in the control of mild to moderate hypertension as an adjunct to thiazides. Captopril, when administered in combination with allopurinol or procainamide, leads to Stevens–Johnson syndrome. It decreases the bronchial secretions leading to a dry persistent cough.

21 A False
   B False
   C True
   D True
   E False
Adrenaline causes a rise in blood sugar due to the breakdown of muscle and liver glycogen and is found to increase the body's total oxygen consumption by 30%.

22 A False
   B True
   C False
   D False
   E False

23 A True
   B True
   C False
   D True
   E False
Procainamide is effective in the control of ventricular arrhythmias following myocardial infarction. It is contraindicated in heart block, hypertension and heart failure. The maximum IV dose is 1 g.

24 Methyldopa
A Causes a marked fall in blood pressure during exercise
B Acts as a false neurotransmitter
C Acts on the Alpha receptors in the hypothalamus
D Side-effects include granulocytopenia
E The D-isomer of methyldopa inhibits dopa decarboxylase activity

25 Phenoxybenzamine
A Is a haloalkylamine
B Its peak effect is attained within 10 min
C Decreases peripheral resistance
D Increases renal blood flow
E Has a high lipid solubility

26 Verapamil
A Prevents entry of calcium through slow channels
B Prevents repolarization of the cell membrane
C Increases sodium entry
D Antagonizes the opening of the fast sodium channel
E Enhances potassium efflux

27 Dopexamine
A Is used in the treatment of high cardiac output failure
B Acts by arterial vasodilation
C Is a $\beta 1$-adrenergic agonist
D Causes bronchodilation
E Is bound to plasma proteins

24 A True
B True
C True
D True
E False
Methyldopa provides an alternative substrate to dopa and is converted to α-methylnoradrenaline which replaces the normal neurotransmitter. The L isomer of methyldopa inhibits dopa decarboxylase activity.

25 A True
B False
C True
D False
E True
The peak effect of phenoxybenzamine is seen in 1 h following IV injection. It increases the cardiac output with a fall in peripheral resistance. It has no effect on the renal blood flow in normovolaemic patients, but causes a fall in hypotensive patients.

26 A True
B False
C False
D False
E False
Verapamil is a synthetic papaverine derivative with antihypertensive and antianginal action. It decreases the influx of calcium ions into vascular smooth muscle and myocardial cells by competitive blockade of cell membrane slow calcium ion channels.

27 A False
B True
C False
D True
E False
Dopexamine is used in the treatment of low cardiac output failure and acute heart failure. It acts by arterial vasodilatation, positive inotropism and renal arterial vasodilatation. It inhibits uptake of noradrenaline and has potent β2-adrenergic agonist activity. Dopexamine is 40% bound to red blood cells and has a volume of distribution between 317 and 446 ml/kg.

28 Diltiazem

A Increases myocardial oxygen demand
B Acts by dose-dependent inhibition of slow calcium channels
C Is a peripheral vasodilator
D Causes vasoconstriction
E Causes bradycardia in association with β blockers

29 Enalapril

A Is an amide
B Acts as an angiotensin-converting enzyme inhibitor
C Causes a fall in cardiac output
D Increases plasma renin activity
E Increases glomerular filtration rate

28 A False
   B True
   C True
   D False
   E True
   Diltiazem is a benzothiapine (not benzodiazepine) which acts by dose-dependent inhibition of the slow calcium current in normal cardiac tissue. It increases myocardial oxygen supply and decreases myocardial oxygen demand by coronary vasodilatation. As it also causes peripheral vasodilatation, diltiazem decreases both systemic and pulmonary vascular resistance and increases the cardiac output due to a reduction in after load. Diltiazem prevents bronchoconstriction due to inhaled histamine and causes a reduction in lower oesophageal pressure in patients with achalasia.

29 A False
   B True
   C False
   D True
   E False
   Enalapril is an ester of Enalaprilat. It acts as an angiotensin-converting enzyme inhibitor and thus prevents the formation of angiotensin II from angiotensin I. The adult oral dose is 5–40 mg daily. It causes a fall in blood pressure by decreasing the systemic vascular resistance by acting predominantly on arteries and arterioles. Cardiac output increases only in the presence of heart failure otherwise there is no change. Enalapril causes an increase in renal blood flow without altering glomerular filtration rate. It is 50% protein bound in the plasma and is absorbed effectively when given orally. Enalapril is a pro-drug which is converted in the liver by hydrolysis to its active form Enalaprilat.

30 Enoximone
- A Is an imidazoline derivative
- B Acts by inhibiting Type II phosphodiesterase
- C Causes a fall in pulmonary capillary wedge pressure
- D Increases myocardial oxygen consumption
- E Has little effect on plasma renin activity

31 Coronary circulation
- A During isometric ventricular relaxation the blood flow in the left coronary artery is decreased
- B At rest the coronary blood flow is 100–200 ml/min
- C Coronary artery blood flow is directly proportional to the myocardial oxygen consumption in the normal range
- D Bradycardia causes a rise in coronary blood flow
- E Stimulation of the stellate ganglion does not affect coronary blood flow

32 Cardiac output
- A Falls with moderate changes in environmental temperature
- B Its regulation due to changes in cardiac muscle fibre length is sometimes called heterometric regulation
- C Increases up to 700% during exercise
- D Histamine has no effect
- E Is changed in pyrexia

30 A True
B False
C True
D False
E True
Enoximone is an imidazoline derivative which acts by inhibiting type IV phosphodiesterase, the enzyme which is responsible for the breakdown of cyclic AMP. It has a positive inotropic action and causes an increase in cardiac output and a fall in pulmonary vascular resistance, wedge pressure and systemic vascular resistance. It has no effect on myocardial oxygen consumption and plasma renin activity. It is used in the treatment of acute or chronic heart failure.

31 A False
B False
C True
D False
E False
Blood flow in the left coronary artery is decreased during isometric left ventricular contraction. At rest the coronary blood flow is 60–80 ml/min per 100 g of tissue. Stimulation of stellate ganglion causes tachycardia, hypertension and increased myocardial contractility.

32 A False
B True
C True
D False
E True
The volume of blood pumped by each ventricle per minute is called the cardiac output. It is also the volume of blood flowing through either systemic or the pulmonary circulation per minute. Cardiac output is the product of heart rate and stroke volume. Heart rate is sensitive to adrenaline, changes in body temperature and plasma electrolytes. Stroke volume is the volume of blood ejected by each ventricle during each contraction. Change in stroke volume is produced by either a change in end-diastolic volume or a change in the magnitude of sympathetic nervous system.

33 Fetal circulation
A 30% of the fetal cardiac output goes through the placenta
B Blood in the umbilical vein has the same saturation as the arterial blood of the adult
C Blood entering the heart from the inferior vena cava is diverted directly to the left atrium via the patent foramen ovale
D Blood from the superior vena cava enters the pulmonary artery via the right ventricle
E The oxygen saturation of blood in the umbilical arteries is 60%

34 Law of Laplace
A States that the pressure in a distensible hollow sphere is directly proportional to the tension in the wall divided by the radius of the sphere $P = 2T/\pi$
B In the human aorta the tension at high pressures is 170 000 dynes/cm
C In the vena cava the tension is 21 000 dynes/cm
D The radius of curvature of an alveolus increases during inspiration
E The less the radius of a blood vessel, the less is the tension in the vessel wall necessary to balance the distending pressure

35 Arterial pressure
A In an upright position the mean pressure in a large artery in the head (50 cm above the heart) is 60 mmHg when the pressure at the heart level is 100 mmHg
B Mean pressure is the sum of diastolic pressure plus half of the pulse pressure
C Falls rapidly in small arteries and arterioles
D Blood pressure falls rapidly to about 5 mmHg at the end of arterioles
E When a blood vessel is narrowed the velocity of flow in this narrowed portion is decreased

36 Diastolic hypertension is seen in:
A Conn's syndrome
B Addison's disease
C Phaeochromocytoma
D Polycystic disease
E Women on oral contraceptives

33 A False
    B False
    C True
    D True
    E True
Some 55% of the fetal cardiac output goes through the placenta
and the blood in the umbilical vein is 80% saturated as compared
with 98% in the arterial blood in the adult.

34 A True
    B False
    C True
    D True
    E True
The pressure measured is the transmural pressure which is
expressed as dynes/sq.cm, whilst tension is expressed as dynes per
cm. The tension in the human aorta is 170 000 dynes/cm at normal
pressures.

35 A True
    B False
    C True
    D True
    E False
The pressure in any vessel above the heart level is decreased by the
effect of gravity. It is the product of the density of blood,
acceleration due to gravity (980 cm/s per s) and the vertical
distance above or below the heart (0.77 mmHg/cm at the density of
the normal blood).

36 A True
    B False
    C True
    D True
    E True
Diastolic hypertension is seen in Cushing's disease rather than in
Addison's disease.

37 Pulse pressure
A Is the difference between systolic and diastolic pressure
B Large stroke volume causes a fall
C There is no change in patients with fever
D Is greatest in patients with aortic regurgitation
E Is abnormal in old age

38 Arterioles
A Are dilated by adrenaline in skeletal muscle
B Hypoxia causes vasoconstriction
C Locally released serotonin causes vasodilatation
D Local axon reflex improves the blood flow
E Kinin-like peptide is one of the causes of migraine

39 Coronary circulation
A Shows autoregulation
B Hypotension causes coronary vasoconstriction
C Injection of adrenaline in the coronary arteries causes vasodilatation
D Left ventricular blood flow is increased during tachycardia
E Coronary blood flow is increased in patients with congestive heart failure

37 A True
    B False
    C True
    D True
    E True

In old age the distensibility of arteries is decreased due to arteriosclerosis, hence an abnormal pulse pressure.

38 A True
    B False
    C False
    D True
    E True

Locally released serotonin causes vasoconstriction and the local axon reflex improves the blood flow due to relay of afferent impulses to the sensory nerves of the arterioles.

39 A True
    B False
    C True
    D False
    E False

Hypotension causes vasodilatation due to a reflex increase in adrenergic stimulation. Coronary flow occurs during diastole and in tachycardia the diastolic period is shortened, leading to decreased flow.
In congestive heart failure the venous pressure rises and by reducing effective coronary perfusion pressure, decreases the coronary blood flow.

40 Venous circulation
A The pressure in the venules is 12–18 cmH$_2$O
B Venous pressure rises by 0.77 mmHg for each centimetre below the right atrium
C Central venous pressure (CVP) changes from 2 mmHg during inspiration to 6 mmHg during expiration
D The CVP along the collapsed segments of neck veins is subatmospheric
E Five ml of air injected intravenously can lead to air embolism

41 Cardiac output
A Decreases in metabolic acidosis
B Decreases by 30% upon changing from recumbent to upright position
C Fast atrial fibrillation does not cause any difference in cardiac output
D Infusion of sodium bicarbonate increases cardiac output by 100%
E Ethyl alcohol causes a rise in output

42 Haemorrhage and haemorrhagic shock
A Results in increased thoracic pumping
B Causes increased activity in the arterial baroreceptors
C Reticular formation is stimulated
D Oxygen-carrying capacity is unchanged
E Filtration fraction is decreased

40 A False
    B True
    C False
    D False
    E True

The pressure in the venules is 12–18 mmHg which falls to 5.5 mmHg in large veins outside the thorax. The rise and fall of venous pressure is of the same degree above or below the right atrium. CVP changes from 6 mmHg during inspiration to 2 mmHg during quiet expiration. The neck veins collapse above the point where the venous pressure is zero and the pressure along the segments is zero rather than subatmospheric. Even a small amount of air lodges in the small blood vessels and stops the blood flow due to an increased resistance against the blood flow.

41 A False
    B True
    C False
    D True
    E True

There is no change in cardiac output in patients with metabolic acidosis, and in patients with fast atrial fibrillation the output may drop by as much as 50%.

42 A True
    B False
    C True
    D False
    E False

An increase in thoracic pumping is a compensatory reaction. The baroreceptors are stretched to a lesser degree with an increased sympathetic outflow as an immediate compensation. Circulating catecholamines stimulate reticular formation making some patients restless and apprehensive. The oxygen-carrying capacity is decreased due to the loss of red blood cells. The filtration fraction (GFR/renal plasma flow) is increased, the reason being that although GFR is decreased, the renal plasma flow is decreased considerably.

43 Cardiac reflexes
A *Mayer waves* are the cyclic activity in efferent discharges from the chemoreceptors to the vasomotor centre
B *Traube–Hering waves* are variations in the blood pressure synchronized with respiration
C A rise in intracranial pressure is associated with a rise in systemic arterial pressure
D *Bainbridge reflex* is a response to a local stretch
E Injection of veratridine into the coronary artery supplying the left ventricle causes hypertension, hyperventilation and tachycardia

44 2,3-Diphosphoglycerate (2,3-DPG) levels
A Are increased by methylprednisolone
B Are decreased during pregnancy
C Are increased in the presence of growth hormone
D Are increased by hypoxia
E Are increased by hypercarbia

45 Pulmonary circulation
A Pulmonary vascular resistance is 105 dynes/cm^2
B Pulmonary capillary wedge pressure reflects mean pressure in the right atrium
C 5% oxygenated pulmonary venous blood is diluted by unoxygenated bronchial venous blood
D Pulmonary arterial pressure falls during inspiration
E Infusion of acetylcholine causes pulmonary vasoconstriction

46 Total peripheral resistance is increased in:
A Haemorrhage
B Changing from supine to a standing position
C Hypertension
D Lifting a heavy load
E Strenuous running

43 A False
  B True
  C True
  D False
  E False
Mayer waves are the afferent discharges which are conveyed to the vasomotor centre. *Cushing reflex* involves hypertension associated with a rise in intracranial pressure. *Bainbridge reflex* is a true reflex as rapid infusion of blood or saline produces a rise in heart rate if the initial rate was low. *Bezold–Jarisch reflex* (following injection of veratridine) consists of hypotension, apnoea and bradycardia.

44 A True
  B False
  C True
  D True
  E False
2,3-Diphosphoglycerate (DPG), which is produced by the RBCs during glycolysis, binds reversibly with haemoglobin, causing it to have a lower affinity for oxygen. The effect of increased 2,3-DPG is to shift the oxyhaemoglobin dissociation curve to the right. 2,3-DPG levels are increased with hypoxia and high altitudes.

45 A True
  B False
  C False
  D True
  E True
Pulmonary capillary wedge pressure reflects mean pressure in the left atrium. 1–2% of dilution occurs due to the free communication between pulmonary and bronchial systems.

46 A True
  B True
  C False
  D False
  E False
The total systemic resistance is increased in subjects changing from supine to a standing position because of a fall in pressure in the carotid sinus or aortic arch.

47 T wave of the electrocardiogram occurs:
A   During the beginning of the refractory period
B   During the depolarization of the heart
C   During atrial systole
D   During the repolarization of the ventricle
E   During the first heart sound

48 Basal metabolic rate (BMR)
A   Is low in temperate climates
B   Is high in children
C   Depressed patients have normal BMR
D   In an adult male is $60\,kcal/m^2$ per h
E   Is expressed as a percentage

49 Reflexes from heart and lungs
A   Bainbridge reflex consists of raised venous pressure and bradycardia following intravenous infusion of saline
B   Bezold–Jarisch reflex involves reflex cardiac slowing, hypotension and apnoea
C   Volume receptors are located in the right atrium
D   Lung inflation reduces sympathetic tone in the skin
E   Respiratory sinus arrhythmia occurs due to sympathetic activity

47 A False
   B False
   C False
   D True
   E False

At the beginning of the refractory period, depolarization of the heart occurs during QRS complex in the ECG. Atrial systole occurs during PR interval and the first heart sound occurs during QRS complex and ends before the beginning of T wave.

48 A False
   B True
   C False
   D False
   E True

BMR is low in tropical climates and in patients who are depressed. In an adult male the BMR is $40\,kcal/m^2$ per h. A value of $+65$ means BMR is 65% above the standard for sex and age.

49 A False
   B True
   C False
   D True
   E False

Bainbridge reflex consists of rise in venous pressure and tachycardia after the infusion of saline, which is due to stretch on the receptors present on the right atrium. The receptors for Bezold–Jarisch reflex are located within the heart or coronary arteries. Volume receptors are located on the left atrium and they help in regulating the blood volume. Respiratory sinus arrhythmia occurs due to waxing and waning of vagal efferent activity in phase with periodic respiratory centre discharge.

50 Osmotic pressure
A   Of a solution varies with the number of molecules in a solution
B   Liver acts as an osmoreceptor
C   On drinking plain tap water the osmotic pressure of the extracellular water (ECW) increases
D   Osmotic pressure of ECW increases in resting supine position
E   Serum sodium concentration varies the osmotic pressure of the ECW proportionately

51 Skeletal muscle and circulation
A   α-adrenergic receptors control muscle blood flow
B   During exercise, sympathetic stimulation of the arterioles is exaggerated
C   The difference in muscle blood flow between man and cat is due to the proportion of red and white fibres in the muscle
D   Bradykinin causes vasodilatation
E   In an athlete, a decrease in blood flow to the skeletal muscle and myocardium is required for adequate muscle perfusion

52 A splitting of second heart sound is due to:
A   A delay in closure of aortic valve
B   A delay in closure of tricuspid valve
C   A delay in closure of mitral valve
D   A delay in closure of pulmonary valve
E   Atrial systole

53 Approximate distribution of blood in vascular system
A   Heart during systole contains 360 ml
B   Pulmonary arteries carry 130 ml
C   Large veins carry 2300 ml
D   Aorta and large arteries carry 300 ml
E   Pulmonary veins carry 2.6% of whole blood

50 A True
  B True
  C False
  D False
  E True

When water is absorbed from the gastrointestinal tract, afferent impulses reach the liver via the splanchnic circulation. From here, second-order impulses are sent to the hypothalamus via the vagus nerve, thus regulating the intake of water from the gastrointestinal tract. On drinking plain tap water the osmotic pressure of the extracellular water (ECW) decreases because of the dilution of ECW. In the resting supine position and cool temperatures there is a decreased secretion of ADH, consequently leading to a fall in osmotic pressure.

51 A True
  B False
  C True
  D True
  E True

During exercise, the sympathetic stimulation of the arterioles is diminished by the effects of vasodilator mechanisms. Red muscles have double the resting blood flow as compared with the white muscles.

52 A False
  B False
  C False
  D True
  E False

During atrial systole, fourth heart sound occurs.

53 A False
  B True
  C False
  D True
  E False

The blood content in the heart during diastole contains 360 ml. Large veins carry 900 ml, whereas small veins carry 2300 ml. Pulmonary veins carry about 4% (200 ml) of the blood in the vascular system.

54 Oxygen availability
A Is increased by a rise in haemoglobin content
B Shivering increases the oxygen requirement
C Is increased following a drop in cardiac output
D With hypothermia (at 30°C), oxygen requirement is decreased by 40%
E Carboxyhaemoglobin lowers the oxygen availability

55 Viscosity and resistance
A Blood flow varies directly with the viscosity of blood
B Viscosity depends on the percentage of the volume of blood occupied by RBCs
C In anaemia, peripheral resistance is increased
D In spherocytosis there is a marked increase in the viscosity of blood
E Rise in plasma immunoglobulin causes a fall in the viscosity

56 Duration of cardiac action potential
A Duration of systole is 0.3 s
B Relative refractory period lasts for 0.05 s
C Duration of diastole is 0.6 s
D Each cardiac cycle lasts for 0.8 s
E Action potential lasts for 0.3 s

57 Events of cardiac cycle
A During protodiastole there is a rapid drop in intraventricular pressure
B Diastasis marks the onset of ventricular contraction
C During isovolumetric contraction, semilunar valves are open
D There is a peak intraventricular pressure during reduced ejection phase
E During isovolumetric relaxation, atrioventricular valves close

54 A True
  B True
  C False
  D True
  E True
Oxygen available/min = haemoglobin content + plasma concentration x cardiac output. It is increased following a rise in cardiac output.

55 A False
  B True
  C False
  D True
  E False
Blood flow varies inversely and resistance directly with the viscosity of the blood. In large vessels an increase in the haematocrit causes an increase in the viscosity. Similarly the viscosity is increased in spherocytosis due to the abnormal rigidity of red blood cells. In anaemia the peripheral resistance is decreased which is partly due to a decrease in the viscosity.

56 A False
  B True
  C False
  D True
  E False
Duration of cardiac action potential varies as follows: systole 0.27 s, diastole 0.53 s and the action potential 0.25 s.

57 A True
  B False
  C True
  D True
  E False
Diastasis marks the onset of atrial contraction. During isometric relaxation the atrioventricular valves open.

58 Circulation in organs
A 70% of splanchnic blood flow reaches the liver via the hepatic artery
B The emptying of splenic blood into circulation is under sympathetic control
C Hepatic arterial flow remains constant when the perfusion pressure is varied
D 30% of total cardiac output passes through both kidneys
E In a supine exercising subject, the renal blood flow is unchanged

59 Cardiac output
A During muscular exercise, myocardial contractility is increased
B Frank–Starling mechanism plays a role in transplanted hearts
C Decreased peripheral resistance facilitates venous return
D Trained athletes have a lower heart rate
E Untrained athletes have a high end-systolic ventricular volume

60 In a Valsalva manoeuvre
A Distension of facial and neck veins occurs
B There is an abolition of intrathoracic pressure
C A positive intrathoracic pressure is developed
D Is used to detect autonomic insufficiency
E There is a forced expiration against open glottis

58 A False
   B True
   C True
   D False
   E True
Some 30% of the blood reaches the liver via the hepatic artery and
70% via the portal vein from the stomach, intestines, spleen and
pancreas. Hepatic arterial flow possesses the property of
autoregulation. About 20% of the cardiac output passes through
both kidneys in normal resting state. The renal blood flow is
unchanged in a supine exercising person as compared with an
upright exercising person where renal blood flow diminishes.

59 A True
   B True
   C False
   D True
   E False
Transplanted hearts increase their output during exercise in the
absence of cardiac innervation through Frank–Starling mechanism.
An increase in peripheral resistance facilitates venous return.
Trained athletes, as compared with untrained, have a high end-
systolic ventricular volume and greater stroke volume at rest.

60 A True
   B True
   C True
   D True
   E False
Valsalva manoeuvre is forced expiration against a closed glottis. At
the onset of straining, the blood pressure rises because of the rise
in intrathoracic pressure. It then falls as the high intrathoracic
pressure decreases. The fall in arterial blood pressure and pulse
pressure inhibit the baroreceptors, causing tachycardia and a rise
in peripheral resistance. After the glottis is opened and the
intrathoracic pressure returns to normal, the cardiac output returns
to normal but the peripheral vessels continue to remain
constricted. The blood pressure thus rises above normal which in
turn stimulates the baroreceptors, causing bradycardia and a drop
in blood pressure to normal levels.

61 Electrocardiogram
A Lead I = $VF - VR$
B Lead II = $VL - VR$
C Lead III = $VF - VL$
D Kirchhoff's second law states that the sum of absolute potentials recorded at right arm, left arm, left leg would be equal to zero
E Precordial lead VI displays a small R wave due to septal activation

62 Adrenergic receptors
A Alpha receptors, when stimulated causes coronary dilatation
B Stimulation of Beta-receptors causes contraction of splenic capsule
C Stimulation of Beta-receptors causes lipolysis
D Beta-receptors situated in the skeletal muscle cause vasoconstriction
E Alpha-receptor stimulation inhibits insulin secretion

63 Venous pressure
A Falls during IPPV
B In Valsalva manoeuvre it is increased
C Is increased rising from supine position
D Falls during exercise
E In the standing position, there is a negative pressure in the sagittal sinus

61 A False
   B False
   C True
   D True
   E True
   Lead I $= VL - VR$; Lead II $= VF - VR$.
   In Kirchhoff's second law $VR + VL + VLF = 0$.
   Precordial lead VI displays a small R wave due to activation of septum from left to right.

62 A False
   B False
   C True
   D False
   E True
   Stimulation of α-receptors causes coronary vasoconstriction and contraction of the splenic capsule. Stimulation of β-receptors causes vasodilatation.

63 A True
   B True
   C False
   D False
   E True
   The venous pressure rises in Valsalva manoeuvre due to impediment of blood flow into the right atrium. It is also increased during exercise as a great amount of blood enters from the arterial side. In a standing position, the veins are not collapsable and there is a hydrostatic pressure difference between the top and the base of the skull.

64 Cardiac performance
A An upright posture has little effect on the end-diastolic filling pressure
B Thoracic pump increases end-diastolic volume
C Pericardial effusion increases end-diastolic volume
D Atrial contraction contributes to 20–30% of ventricular filling
E Unidirectional venous valves promote venous return

65 Of the cardiac output at rest in a 70 kg male
A Splanchnics receive 1200 ml/min
B Heart receives 250 ml/min
C Muscles receive 1400 ml/min
D Kidneys receive 1100 ml/min
E Skin receives 500 ml/min

66 Catecholamines
A Adrenaline is metabolized by hydroxylation
B Catechol o-methyltransferase (COMT) catalyses methylation reaction
C Monoamine oxidase (MAO) catalyses oxidation
D COMT is found in adrenergic nerve endings
E Vanillylmandelic acid (VMA) is the metabolite present in the urine

64 A False
B True
C False
D True
E True
An upright posture reduces intrathoracic and end-diastolic filling pressure. The intrathoracic pressure is negative during spontaneous ventilation and constitutes a thoracic pump. Pericardial effusion interferes with ventricular distensibility and decreases the end-diastolic volume.

65 A False
B True
C False
D True
E True
The splanchnics receive 1400 ml/min, muscles 1200 ml/min.

66 A False
B True
C True
D False
E True
Adrenaline and noradrenaline are metabolized to biologically inactive products by oxidation and methylation. Catechol *o*-methyltransferase (COMT) is widely distributed, with high concentration in the liver and kidneys, but not in the adrenergic nerve endings.

3 Respiratory system

1 Theophyllines
  A Stimulate the spinal cord
  B Cause a fall in blood pressure
  C Cause a fall in cerebral blood flow
  D Depress the motility of the large intestine
  E Increase the coagulation time

2 Disodium cromoglycate
  A Is effective by parenteral route
  B Prevents mast cell degranulation
  C Is an antihistamine
  D Inhalation of fine powder occasionally causes bronchospasm
  E Half-life is 1 h

3 Doxapram
  A Acts on the respiratory centre
  B Acts within 20–40 s after IV injection
  C Causes bradycardia
  D At higher doses increases the tidal volume
  E Decreases gastrointestinal tone

1 A True
  B False
  C True
  D True
  E False
Theophyllines cause a rise in cardiac output due to a direct action on the myocardium. They shorten the coagulation time.

2 A False
  B True
  C False
  D True
  E True
Disodium cromoglycate is effective by inhalation or by topical application to the nasal mucosa.

3 A True
  B True
  C False
  D False
  E False
Doxapram is a pyrrolidinone derivative. When given IV it acts in 20–40 seconds; its peak effect being seen in 1–2 min with a duration of action of 5–12 min. Doxapram causes an increase in cardiac output due to an increase in the stroke volume. It also causes an increase in blood pressure, heart rate. At low doses, doxapram increases minute volume by increasing the tidal volume and at high doses causes an increase in respiratory rate.

4 Ipratropium
A Is a derivative of atropine
B Is effective when given orally and IV
C Causes tachycardia and hypertension after inhalation
D Causes mydriasis
E Crosses blood/brain barrier

5 Salbutamol
A Is a sympatholytic agent
B Acts as a uterine relaxant
C Increases intracellular cyclic AMP concentration
D Is effective when given IM
E Increases peripheral vascular resistance

6 Terbutaline
A Is a β-adrenergic agonist
B Decreases the function of the neonatal lung
C Causes hyperinsulinaemia
D Is used in complicated preterm labour
E Is an alcohol

4 A True
  B True
  C False
  D True
  E False

Ipratropium is a synthetic quaternary ammonium compound which is a derivative of atropine. It causes bronchodilatation by competitive inhibition of cholinergic receptors on bronchial smooth muscle. Ipratropium has no effect on cardiovascular system when administered by inhalation method, but causes tachycardia and hypertension when given IV. It causes mydriasis and does not cross the blood/brain barrier. When given orally in large doses it causes a decrease in salivation and gastric secretion.

5 A False
  B True
  C True
  D True
  E False

Salbutamol is a sympathomimetic amine which causes bronchodilatation and uterine relaxation. It acts by stimulation of membrane-bound adenyl cyclase to increase intracellular cyclic AMP concentration. In high doses salbutamol has a positive inotropic and chronotropic effect. At lower doses it causes a fall in blood pressure by decreasing the peripheral vascular resistance. The adult oral dose is 2–4 mg 6–8 hourly, the IM dose being 0.5 mg 4 hourly. Salbutamol is given in the inhaler form, one to two metered puffs of 200–400 mcg every 6–8 hours. Salbutamol decreases the tone of gravid uterus and decreases the plasma potassium concentration.

6 A True
  B False
  C True
  D False
  E True

Terbutaline is an alcoholic compound and a β-adrenergic agonist. In high doses it has a positive inotropic and chronotropic effect. It relaxes uterine musculature when given in the antepartum period. Terbutaline stimulates the release of surfactant material improving the function of the neonatal lung. Following the administration of terbutaline, it can cause hypoglycaemia and hypokalaemia as a result of hyperinsulinaemia. The adult oral dose is 2.5–5 mg 8 hourly, the IM, IV dose being 0.25–0.5 mg twice a day. The dose by inhalation route is 0.25–0.5 mcg every 4 hours.

7 Respiration
A Active and passive movements of joints stimulate respiration
B Sneezing involves keeping the glottis open
C During hiccup the glottis is kept open
D Hyperventilation during shock is mediated by baroreceptors
E Yawning increases the venous return

8 Shunt
A Is defined as the blood which enters the arterial system without passing through unventilated areas of the lung
B Can be due to coronary venous blood which drains into the cavity of the right ventricle through Thebesian veins
C Oxygen content of end-capillary blood can be calculated from alveolar PO_2 and oxygen dissociation curve
D Administration of 100% oxygen relieves the shunt
E Causes a rise in PCO_2

9 Ventilation
A Intrapleural pressure is more negative at the bottom of the lung than at the top of the lung
B At high volumes the lungs become stiffer
C Base of the lung has a large resting volume
D Apex of the lung has a small change in volume on inspiration
E Airway closure occurs at low lung volumes in young people

7 A True
   B True
   C False
   D False
   E True
Sneezing is an expiratory effort with a continuously open glottis.
Hiccup is a spasmodic contraction of the diaphragm which produces
an inspiration during which the glottis suddenly closes.
Hyperventilation during shock is mediated by the chemoreceptors
which are stimulated by stagnant hypoxia and acidosis.

8 A False
   B False
   C True
   D False
   E False
Blood passes through the ventilated areas rather than the
unventilated areas. Coronary venous blood drains into the left
ventricle. Administration of 100% oxygen does not relieve the shunt
because the shunted blood which bypasses the ventilated alveoli are
not exposed to high alveolar PO_2. There is a fall in PCO_2 due to
chemoreceptor stimulation.

9 A False
   B True
   C False
   D True
   E True
The intrapleural pressure is less negative ($-2.5\,cmH_2O$) at the
bottom as compared with the top ($-10\,cmH_2O$) due to the weight
of the lungs. The base of the lung has a low resting volume as the
expanding pressure at the base of the lung is small. Airway closure
occurs in elderly people at high lung volumes due to the loss of
elastic recoil.

18 2,3-Diphosphoglycerate (2,3-DPG)
A   Is formed from 3-phosphoglyceraldehyde
B   Binds to the β-chains of the oxyhaemoglobin
C   Thyroid hormone has no effect on 2,3-DPG
D   Rises during exercise in trained athletes
E   Is increased in chronic hypoxia

19 Alveolar dead space
A   Is that part of inspired gas which passes anatomical dead space but does not take part in the exchange
B   Is less in the upright position than in the supine position
C   Is decreased following pulmonary embolism
D   Clamping of the pulmonary artery does not affect alveolar dead space
E   Increases in patients undergoing spontaneous general anaesthesia as compared with controlled ventilation

20 Pulmonary circulation
A   The mean arterial pressure (MPAP) is 8 mmHg
B   Amount of blood in the pulmonary circulation is between 0.5 and 1.0 l
C   Pulmonary blood volume increases from erect to supine position
D   Barbiturate administration causes a rise in pulmonary blood volume
E   Pulmonary vascular pressures are one-sixth of the systemic arterial pressure

18 A   True
B   False
C   False
D   False
E   True
2,3-DPG is derived from 3-phosphoglyceraldehyde which is a product of glycolysis via the Embden–Meyerhof pathway. One mol of *deoxygenated* blood only binds to one mol of 2,3-DPG. Thyroid hormones, androgens and growth hormone increase the concentration of 2,3-DPG and P50. Exercise produces a rise in 2,3-DPG within 60 min in untrained athletes. It is increased in chronic hypoxia, thus facilitating the delivery of oxygen to the tissues.

19 A   True
B   False
C   False
D   False
E   True
Alveolar dead space is increased in the upright position following pulmonary embolism and after the clamping of the pulmonary artery.

20 A   False
B   True
C   True
D   False
E   True
The mean pulmonary artery pressure is 15 mmHg and the amount of blood in the pulmonary circulation is about 10–20% of the total blood volume. Pulmonary blood volume increases by about 27% when subject changes from erect to supine position. Barbiturates cause a fall in blood volume by about 340 ml.

21 Functions of the lung
  A   Inactivates prostaglandin E
  B   Transfers angiotensin I unaffected through the lung
  C   The enzyme which inactivates bradykinin activates
       angiotensin I
  D   Secretes IgG
  E   Plays a role in the coagulation of blood

22 Anatomical dead space (ADS)
  A   Extending the neck decreases ADS
  B   Sitting position increases ADS
  C   Pneumonectomy results in an increase in ADS
  D   Hypoventilation causes a marked reduction in ADS
  E   Volume of ADS is equal to the weight of subject in kilograms

23 Ventilation/perfusion
  A   Respiratory exchange ratio is higher at the apex than at the
       base
  B   During exercise the base of the lung has a high O_2 uptake
  C PCO_2 levels are normal
  D   Ventilation/perfusion ratio increases down the lung
  E   Ventilation/perfusion ratio reaches infinity when there is an
       obstruction to the blood flow

24 Respiratory muscles
  A   Accessory muscles contract during exercise and elevate the first
       two ribs
  B   External intercostal muscles slope downward and forward
  C   Diaphragm is supplied by C2 and C3 nerves
  D   Expiratory muscles are rectus, transversus abdominus
  E   The internal intercostal muscles increase the thoracic volume

21 A True
   B False
   C True
   D False
   E True
Angiotensin I is converted to angiotensin II in the lung which is 50 times more active. The lung secretes IgA immunoglobulin in the bronchial mucous which contributes to its defence against infection. Lung also plays an important role in the coagulation of blood via mast cells containing heparin in the interstitium.

22 A False
   B True
   C False
   D True
   E False
The volume of ADS is equal to the weight of subject in pounds.

23 A True
   B False
   C True
   D False
   E True
The respiratory exchange ratio is high at the apex because the difference in the CO_2 output is less and is closely related to ventilation. During exercise the apex of the lung has a larger share of oxygen uptake due to uniform distribution of blood flow. The ventilation/perfusion ratio decreases down the lung.

24 A True
   B True
   C False
   D True
   E False
The accessory muscles elevate the first two ribs along with sternomastoid, thus raising the sternum. When the external intercostals contract, the ribs are pulled forward and upward causing an increase in lateral and anteroposterior diameter of the thorax. The diaphragm is supplied by the phrenic nerve which is derived from C3, 4, 5. The other expiratory muscles are internal and external oblique. The internal intercostals decrease the thoracic volume by pulling the ribs downwards and inward during active expiration.

25 Oxyhaemoglobin dissociation curve
A Increased temperature shifts it to the left
B Citrate phosphate dextrose blood decreases the rate of 2,3-DPG depletion
C Anaemia results in a fall in 2,3-DPG
D High altitude shifts the curve to the right
E Halothane increases P50

26 Carbon dioxide
A CO_2 dissociation curve is bell-shaped
B Is carried in combination with carbamino compounds
C CO_2 is 10 times less soluble than oxygen
D Oxygenation enhances the unloading of CO_2
E Haem combines with CO_2

27 Oxygen-diffusing capacity
A Pulmonary oedema causes little change
B Emphysema reduces the diffusing capacity due to destruction of surfactant
C Is decreased in patients with raised cardiac output
D Is oxygen uptake/(alveolar PO_2 − mean capillary PO_2)
E A reduction in pulmonary capillary blood volume decreases the oxygen-diffusing capacity

25 A False
   B True
   C False
   D True
   E False

In patients with anaemia and at high altitudes, the levels of 2,3-DPG are increased. 2,3-DPG has an increased affinity for haemoglobin, thus increasing the oxygen available to the tissues. Halothane has no effect on P50.

26 A False
   B True
   C False
   D True
   E False

CO_2 dissociation curve is linear in shape. It is 20 times more soluble than O_2 and the mechanism by which oxygenation enhances the unloading of CO_2 is called *Haldane effect*. Globin, and not haem, combines with CO_2 to form carbamino compounds.

27 A False
   B False
   C True
   D True
   E True

Pulmonary oedema causes a fall in oxygen-diffusing capacity because of the increasing length of the diffusion pathway for oxygen within the pulmonary capillaries. Emphysema reduces the diffusing capacity due to the destruction of alveolar septa. Oxygen-diffusing capacity is increased in patients with raised cardiac output due to an increased capillary transit time. A reduction in pulmonary capillary blood volume decreases the oxygen-diffusing capacity due to reduced area of functioning interface.

28 Physiological dead space
  A Is that part of the tidal volume which does not take part in gaseous exchange
  B Increases with age
  C Prolonged inspiration increases physiological dead space
  D Is calculated as: $[V_t(PaCO_2 - PECO_2)/PECO_2]$ – apparatus dead space
  E Intermittent positive-pressure ventilation (IPPV) increases the physiological dead space

29 At altitude
  A The barometric pressure at 18 000 feet (5500 metres) is 380 mmHg
  B Ventilation is increased threefold as a compensation
  C Polycythaemia is a response to hypoxaemia
  D Oxygen dissociation curve is shifted to the left
  E Pulmonary vasoconstriction occurs

30 Oxygen dissociation curve
  A Shows a relation between PO_2, haemoglobin saturation and oxygen capacity
  B Steep lower part of the curve shows large amounts of oxygen can be withdrawn by tissues for a small decrease in capillary PO_2
  C A fall in pH shifts the curve to the right
  D 2,3-DPG shifts the curve to the left
  E Is similar to carbon monoxide dissociation curve

28 A True
B True
C False
D False
E False
Prolonged inspiration decreases physiological dead space (PDS).
PDS is calculated as

$$\frac{V_T(P_{a}CO_2 - P_{E}CO_2)}{P_{a}CO_2} - \text{apparatus dead space}$$

IPPV has no effect on PDS.

29 A True
B False
C True
D False
E True
When a person arrives at a high altitude, he develops transient
'mountain sickness' within 24–48 h and lasting for 4–8 days. It is
characterized by headache, irritability, insomnia, breathlessness,
nausea and vomiting. Pulmonary oedema tends to occur in
individuals who ascent quickly to altitudes above 2500 m.
Respiratory alkalosis occurs as a compensatory mechanism as a
result of acclimatization to altitude. The oxyhaemoglobin
dissociation curve is shifted to left with an increase in 2,3-DPG
and P50. Erythropoietin secretion increases promptly on ascent to
high altitude and then falls over the following 4 days. The
compensatory mechanisms which occur in tissue include increase in
the number of mitochondria and myoglobin level.

30 A False
B True
C True
D False
E True
Oxyhaemoglobin dissociation curve shows a relation between P_{O_2},
haemoglobin saturation and oxygen content. It is similar to carbon
monoxide dissociation curve except the axis of the latter is greatly
compressed.

31 Pressures during respiratory cycle
A Alveolar pressure rises to allow inspiratory flow to occur
B Intrapleural pressure is $-5\,cmH_2O$ before inspiration begins
C Alveolar pressure is positive during expiration
D Fall in intrapleural pressure during inspiration is due to a fall in the elastic recoil
E With forced expiration, the intrapleural pressure exceeds zero

32 Oxygen toxicity
A Is due to free radicals $(O_3{}^-)$
B Is also called Lorraine–Smith effect
C Exposure of 24 h to 2 atm of oxygen produces substernal distress
D Results in alveolar consolidation
E Can cause respiratory arrest

33 Lung volumes and capacities
A The air inspired with a maximal inspiratory effort in excess of tidal volume is inspiratory reserve volume
B Air present in the lungs after a maximal inspiratory effort is the residual volume
C Timed vital capacity is decreased in asthma
D Normal maximal voluntary ventilation is 250–300 l/min
E Vital capacity includes tidal volume, expiratory reserve volume and residual volume

34 In a healthy subject, response to strenuous training is:
A A decrease in the ejection fraction of the ventricles
B A decrease in the maximum dP/dt of the left ventricle
C An increase in the circulation time
D A decrease in A–V oxygen difference
E An increase in the concentration of plasma lactate

31 A False
   B True
   C True
   D False
   E True
Alveolar pressure falls, thus establishing the driving pressure for inspiratory flow. A fall in the intrapleural pressure is due to an increase in the elastic recoil.

32 A True
   B True
   C False
   D False
   E True
Exposure of 10 h to 1 atm of oxygen produces substernal distress. It can also result in alveolar collapse.

33 A True
   B False
   C True
   D False
   E False
Air present in the lungs after a maximal expiratory effort is called the residual volume. Timed vital capacity is also called forced expired volume in 1 second (FEV_1). The normal maximal voluntary ventilation, also called maximal breathing capacity (125–170 l/min) is the largest volume of gas that can be moved into and out of the lu. ·s in 1 min by voluntary effort.

34 A False
   B False
   C False
   D False
   E True
The response to strenuous training consists of an increase in the ejection fraction and an increase in end systolic volume and also an increase in the maximum dP/dt of the left ventricle due to a rise in catecholamines. There is also an increase in A–V oxygen difference and a ninefold rise in the plasma lactate concentration.

35 Surfactant
A Lowers the surface tension in alveoli
B Keeps the alveolus dry
C Its loss causes pulmonary oedema
D Monopalmitoyl-lecithin, a phospholipid, is synthesized in the lung
E Type I cells lining alveoli show osmiophilic lamellar bodies

36 Airway resistance
A Patients with increased airway resistance breathe at low lung volumes
B Smoking increases airway resistance
C Acetylcholine has no action
D Is decreased with helium–oxygen mixture
E Changes in viscosity have an influence on airway resistance

37 Control of ventilation
A Central chemoreceptors respond to changes in H^+ ion concentration
B A change in cerebrospinal fluid pH for a given change in P_{CO_2} is less than in blood
C Peripheral chemoreceptors are situated in the aortic bodies
D Peripheral chemoreceptors respond to changes in arterial P_{O_2}
E Aortic bodies respond to a fall in arterial pH

35 A True
B True
C True
D False
E False
By lowering the surface tension in the alveoli, surfactant reduces the work of expanding it with each breath. It also prevents the transudation of fluid. Dipalmitoyl-lecithin is synthesized in the lungs from the fatty acids. Type II cells lining lung alveoli show osmiophilic lamellated bodies.

36 A False
B True
C False
D True
E False
Patients with increased airway resistance breathe at high lung volumes, thus reducing the airway resistance. Smoking increases the airway resistance by stimulation of receptors in the trachea and large bronchi. Acetylcholine causes bronchoconstriction, thus increasing the resistance. Changes in density and not viscosity have an influence on the airway resistance because the flow is not purely laminar in the medium-sized airways.

37 A True
B False
C True
D True
E False
A change in cerebrospinal fluid pH for a given change in P_{CO_2} is greater than in blood because the former contains less protein than blood with a much lower buffering capacity. Aortic and carotid bodies are the peripheral receptors that are located at the bifurcation of the common carotid arteries. Peripheral chemoreceptors respond to changes in arterial P_{O_2} due to a small arteriovenous difference. In human beings carotid and not aortic bodies respond to a fall in arterial pH.

38 Surfactant
  A Phosphatidyl-dimethylethanolamine is one of the components
  B Is highly soluble
  C Is secreted by the Type I alveolar lining cells
  D Lecithin/sphingomyelin ratio in the amniotic fluid is a measure of the level of lecithin
  E Anaesthesia decreases its action

39 Ventilation/perfusion relationships
  A Blood flow increases more rapidly than ventilation from the bottom to the top of the upright lung
  B When a subject lies supine, the apical and basal blood flows are equal
  C In the lateral position, the anterior region of the lungs are better perfused than the dependent region
  D Uneven distribution of blood flow is caused by the hydrostatic pressure differences within the lung
  E At the base of the lung, the parenchyma is poorly expanded

40 Airway resistance
  A Normal airway resistance is $1-3\,cmH_2O/l$ per s at $0.5\,l/s$ flow rate
  B Is increased in pulmonary oedema
  C Is decreased by acetylcholine
  D Is decreased by atropine
  E Is increased by morphine

38 A True
B False
C False
D True
E False

Phosphatidyl-dimethylethanolamine is one of the constituents of the surfactant, along with lecithin, sphingomyelin and phosphatidylinositol. It is highly insoluble and floats on the surface of the alveolar lining fluid. It is secreted by Type II alveolar lining cells. As the amount of sphingomyelin remains constant, the quantity of lecithin in the amniotic fluid rises sharply late in gestation, hence the measurement of lecithin and sphingomyelin ratio is important. Anaesthesia has no effect on the surfactant.

39 A False
B True
C False
D True
E True

Blood flow increases more rapidly than ventilation from the top to the bottom of the upright lung. The ventilation/perfusion ratio has a high value. In the lateral or supine position, the dependent part (posterior) of the lung has a higher blood flow than the anterior region.

40 A True
B True
C False
D True
E True

Acetylcholine, histamine and irritant gases cause vasoconstriction and an increase in airway resistance, whereas drugs like atropine, isoprenaline, adrenaline and ganglion blockers cause vasodilatation and thus decrease the airway resistance. Pethidine and barbiturates produce little change in the resistance.

41 P50
  A Normal value for adult human blood is 26 mmHg
  B Is decreased by acidosis
  C Fall in P50 indicates low affinity of haemoglobin for oxygen
  D Is increased by high levels of 2,3-DPG
  E Is the tension at which haemoglobin is 50% saturated

42 Decompression sickness
  A During rapid ascent nitrogen is removed rapidly
  B Helium–oxygen mixtures can prevent deep divers' decompression sickness
  C During diving the pressure increases by one atmosphere for every 30 feet of descent
  D The increased density of the gas at depth increases the work of breathing
  E Diver inhales as he ascends

43 Respiratory alkalosis
  A The pH is high
  B CO_2 content is low
  C Chloride concentration is low
  D Serum phosphate is high
  E Serum sodium concentration is high

44 Alveolar pressure
  A Is higher than intrapleural pressure during inspiration
  B Is less negative than intrapleural pressure during expiration
  C Is higher than intrapleural pressure during expiration
  D Is lower than intrapleural pressure during expiration
  E Is lower than intrapleural pressure during inspiration and expiration

41 A True
    B False
    C False
    D True
    E True
P50 is increased by acidosis and a rise in P50 indicates low affinity of haemoglobin for oxygen.

42 A True
    B True
    C False
    D True
    E False
During diving the pressure increases by 1 atm for every 33 feet (not 30 feet) of descent. During ascent, the divers exhale in order to prevent overinflation and rupture of the lungs.

43 A True
    B True
    C False
    D False
    E False
The chloride concentration in respiratory alkalosis is high and the bicarbonate is reciprocally low. The sodium concentration is low due to its increased excretion by the kidneys.

44 A False
    B False
    C True
    D False
    E False
The alveolar pressure is higher (or less negative) than intrapleural pressure during expiration because the surface tension exerted by the liquid lining the alveolar lumen and recoil of alveolar wall increase the pressure.

45 Variations in ventilation
A Upper zones of the lung ventilate better than the lower regions
B In supine volunteers, the lower zones ventilate better than upper zones
C In the lateral position the dependent lung is best ventilated
D Differences in ventilation can be measured using IV radioactive xenon
E Regional differences in ventilation are defined as the change in volume per unit resting volume

46 Response to ventilation
A A reduction in arterial PCO_2 increases the stimulus to ventilation
B Raising the PCO_2 increases the ventilation at any PO_2
C An increase in arterial pH stimulates ventilation
D Arterial pH falls during moderate exercise
E Passive movement of the limbs stimulates ventilation

47 Transfer factor
A Is higher for males than females
B Increases in polycythaemia
C Decreases with higher concentrations of oxygen
D Increases in changes of posture from head-down to upright position
E Is decreased with deep inspiration

45 A False
   B False
   C True
   D False
   E True

The lower zones ventilate better than upper zones and this difference disappears when the subject lies supine. The differences in ventilation can be measured by allowing the subject to inhale radioactive xenon[133] gas.

46 A False
   B True
   C False
   D False
   E True

Reduction in arterial PCO_2 decreases the stimulus to ventilation. A fall in arterial pH stimulates ventilation. The pH remains constant at moderate exercise but falls during heavy exercise due to liberation of lactic acid.

47 A True
   B True
   C True
   D False
   E False

Transfer of gas from the alveoli to blood depends on the diffusion ability of the lung membrane and the rate at which oxygen or carbon dioxide combine with haemoglobin. Diffusing capacity is the process of diffusion across the membrane which separates alveolus from the pulmonary capillary blood, whereas transfer factor describes the whole process. Transfer factor increases with deep inspiration and changing the posture from upright to head-down.

48 Respiratory quotient (RQ)
A Of ethyl alcohol is 0.67
B Is decreased in metabolic acidosis
C Falls following exercise
D RQ of brain is 0.97
E Stomach has a negative RQ during the period of quiescence

49 Pulmonary blood volume
A Is decreased with exercise
B Is increased in patients with mitral stenosis
C Is decreased following meals
D Is increased with age
E Is increased in pulmonary hypertension

50 The following symbols are used in respiratory physiology
A $C\bar{V}O_2$ is the oxygen content of venous blood
B ATPS is the actual temperature pressure saturated
C FiO_2 is the fractional inspired oxygen content
D BTPS is the body temperature pressure saturated
E STPD is standard temperature pressure dry

48 A True
    B False
    C True
    D True
    E False

Respiration quotient (RQ) is the ratio of the volume of CO_2 produced to the volume of O_2 consumed per unit of time. In severe acidosis the RQ may be greater than 1.0 and it tends to fall in respiratory alkalosis. During exercise the RQ reaches 2.00 because of hyperventilation and blowing off of CO_2. During secretion of gastric juice, the stomach has a negative RQ because it takes up more CO_2 from the arterial blood than it puts into the venous blood.

49 A False
    B True
    C True
    D False
    E False

Pulmonary blood volume is increased after exercise and in patients with mitral stenosis, the rise in the latter being due to a rise in pulmonary venous pressure. It is decreased following meals and vasodilatation.

50 A False
    B False
    C False
    D True
    E True

$C\bar{v}O_2$ is the oxygen content of mixed venous blood. ATPS is the ambient temperature pressure saturated. FiO_2 is the fractional inspired oxygen tension.

51 Exercise
  A   In severe exercise, the $PaCO_2$ falls
  B   Oxygen debt is seen during exercise
  C   Tissue PO_2 falls
  D   Oxygen dissociation curve is shifted to the left
  E   The stimulus to ventilation is $PaCO_2$

52 Carbon dioxide production
  A   Increases in hyperthermia
  B   Decreases in obese subjects
  C   Is determined by body mass
  D   Decreases with age
  E   Is decreased in males

53 Lung function tests
  A   Body plethysmograph is used to determine thoracic lung volumes
  B   Debono whistle test indicates the ability to shift air
  C   Maximum expiratory flow rate (MEFR) measures the time to expire 2 l of air after a maximal inspiration
  D   Maximum breathing capacity (MBC) depends on the respiratory excursion only
  E   Timed vital capacity assesses the degree of reversibility of airway obstruction

51 A True
    B True
    C True
    D False
    E False

Pa_{CO_2} falls and Pa_{O_2} rises during exercise due to an increase in ventilation. Oxygen consumption rises maximally with exercise above which blood lactic acid rises. This acid is produced in muscles which cannot keep pace with its utilization, hence oxygen debt occurs. A rise in 2,3-DPG causes a threefold increase in oxygen extraction from each unit of blood. The stimulation to ventilation during exercise is the decreased arterial pH due to lactic acidosis.

52 A True
    B False
    C True
    D True
    E False

Carbon dioxide production increases by 7% for each degree centigrade rise in temperature. It is decreased in old age, and at the age of 70 the values are $88\,ml/m^2$. CO_2 production at the age of 20 years in male is $110\,ml/m^2$ as compared with $96\,ml/m^2$ in females.

53 A True
    B True
    C False
    D False
    E True

Body plethysmograph is also used to measure airway resistance. Along with Snider match test, Debono whistle test is a useful bedside test which requires minimum equipment. In Debono whistle test the patient blows down a wide-bore tube at the end of which is a whistle. In the side of this is an adjustable leak hole. The whistle blows when the rate of airflow through the whistle exceeds a certain value. Maximum breathing capacity of the lungs depends on the size of the respiratory excursion and on the rate at which the lungs can be ventilated.

54 Lung compliance
A   Is related to lung capacity
B   Is decreased in pulmonary oedema
C   Decreases in old age
D   Is decreased with falling lung volumes
E   Is increased in patients with emphysema

55 Lung volumes
A   Exhaled volume of gases following a maximal inspiration is called tidal volume
B   Residual volume falls when the subject rises from a supine position
C   Residual volume is increased to 40% of the total lung capacity in old age
D   Expiratory reserve volume is equal to the residual volume in the upright position
E   Functional residual capacity is the buffer between alveolar ventilation and gas exchanging surface of the lung

56 Carbon dioxide
A   Deoxygenation of the blood increases its ability to carry carbon dioxide
B   Dissolved carbon dioxide obeys Henry's Law
C   In the arterial blood, 60% of carbon dioxide is dissolved in bicarbonate
D   30% of carbon dioxide is present in the A–V difference as carbamino compounds
E   Conversion of carbonic acid into hydrogen and bicarbonate involves carbonic anhydrase

54 A False
    B True
    C False
    D True
    E True

Compliance is defined as the change in lung volume per unit change in airway pressure. The normal value is $0.2 \, l/cmH_2O$). It is greater when measured during deflation than when measured during inflation. Compliance is decreased in pulmonary fibrosis and congestion.

55 A False
    B False
    C True
    D True
    E True

When a subject takes a maximal breath followed by a maximal expiration, the exhaled volume is called vital capacity. Residual volume is the volume of air remaining in the lung after a maximal expiration and is little affected by postural changes. It is increased by 40% in old age due to a decrease in the elastic recoil pressure in the lung. Functional residual capacity minimizes the fluctuations in alveolar gas composition which occurs during tidal breathing.

56 A True
    B True
    C True
    D True
    E False

The increased ability of deoxygenated blood to carry CO_2 is called Haldane effect. Some 60% of the carbon dioxide is dissolved in bicarbonate in the arterial blood and 30% as carbamino compounds and 10% in the dissolved form.

4   Endocrine system

1 **Metformin**
   A   Is metabolized in the liver
   B   Causes ketonuria
   C   Overdose leads to severe lactic acidosis
   D   Has a half-life of 6 h
   E   Can be used in overweight diabetics

2 **Propylthiouracil**
   A   Inhibits peripheral conversion of thyroxine (T_4) and tri-iodothyronine (T_3) quickly
   B   Improvement in thyroid function is noted in a fortnight
   C   Agranulocytosis occurs in less than 1% of the patients
   D   Crosses the placental barrier
   E   Can concentrate in milk

3 **Sulphonylureas**
   A   Chlorpropamide is metabolized in the kidneys
   B   The half-life of tolbutamide is 8 h
   C   Glibenclamide has a half-life of 10–15 h
   D   Chlorpropamide/alcohol flushing is a recessively inherited trait
   E   Sulphonamides potentiate their action

Endocrine system: Answers

1 A False
   B True
   C True
   D False
   E True
Metformin is a biguanide and is used in the treatment of non-insulin-dependent diabetes mellitus. It acts by enhancing the peripheral action of insulin and also by inhibiting the intestinal absorption of glucose and decreasing the peripheral utilization of glucose. The adult dose is 1.5–3 g daily in divided dose. Metformin has a duration of action of 8–12 h. Lactic acidosis can occur as a complication after the use of this drug.

2 A False
   B False
   C True
   D True
   E True
Propylthiouracil is an antithyroid drug which affects the processing of T_4 in peripheral tissues. Propylthiouracil is effective when given orally and has a half-life of 2 h. It crosses the placental barrier.

3 A False
   B True
   C True
   D False
   E True
Sulphonylureas in the presence of glucose increase insulin release, sensitizing the β-cells to glucose. They act by binding to specific receptors that are coupled to increased entry of Ca^{2+} into the β-cells, thus enhancing secretion. Sulphonylureas enhance the effect of insulin in stimulating glucose uptake into muscle and fat cells. The drugs included under sulphonylureas are tolbutamide, acetohexamide, glipizide and glyburide.

4 Ergometrine and oxytocin
A Ergometrine produces slow generalized contraction of the uterus
B Oxytocin is used for induction of labour
C Ergometrine is active for 6 h
D Methylergometrine does not cause long-lasting hypertension
E Causes vomiting due to the effect on chemoreceptor trigger zone

5 Prostaglandins
A Are produced by seminal vesicles
B Are synthesized in the body from saturated fatty acids
C Cyclo-oxygenase catalyses conversion of arachidonic acid to prostaglandin endoperoxides
D Prostaglandin E is a vasodilator
E Prostaglandin F precipitates asthma

6 Insulin preparations
A Action of protamine zinc insulin lasts for 12–18 h
B Neutral insulin has a pH of 7
C Peak action of insulin zinc suspension, crystalline BP is 10–20 h
D The onset of action of isophane insulin is 4 h
E 60–80% of insulin can be lost due to binding to the IV fluid container and tubing

4 A False
   B True
   C False
   D True
   E True
Ergometrine produces faster contraction superimposed on a tonic contraction. Its action lasts for 3 h.
Oxytocin is a naturally occurring polypeptide derived from the posterior lobe of the pituitary gland. It acts by causing uterine contraction. It acts by binding to the receptors on smooth muscle cells and increasing the permeability of the myometrial cell membrane to potassium ions thus increasing the excitability of uterine smooth muscle. Oxytocin also has an antidiuretic effect and causes milk ejection by causing contraction of smooth muscle within the mammary gland. It has a half-life of 1–7 min and is effective when given parenterally.

5 A True
   B False
   C True
   D True
   E True
Prostaglandins form one branch of a large family of endogenous compounds called eicosanoids. These eicosanoids exert profound effects on all cells and tissues and thus provide pharmacological treatment of several diseases. The prostaglandins originate from arachidonic acid, a major compound of mammalian membrane phospholipids. Prostaglandins are synthesized in response to diverse stimuli. They exert their action by binding to specific membrane receptors. Prostaglandin E_1 and prostaglandin E_2 inhibit basal and stimulated gastric acid production and pepsin secretion.

6 A False
   B True
   C True
   D False
   E True
The peak action of protamine zinc insulin is 12–18 h and its duration of action lasts for 24–36 h. The onset of action of isophane insulin is 2 h.

7 Insulin
A Is a polypeptide with four peptide chains
B Its action involves activating the 'second messenger'
C Decreases glucose uptake in the peripheral tissues
D Enhances protein synthesis
E β-cell output of insulin is 40 units/day

8 Biguanides
A Act by stimulating secretion of insulin by the pancreas
B Have a short half-life
C Cause ketonuria
D Are used in juvenile onset diabetes
E Are teratogenic

9 The following are penicillinase resistant:
A Methicillin
B Phenethicillin
C Nafcillin
D Ampicillin
E Carbenicillin

7 A False
  B True
  C False
  D True
  E True
Insulin is a polypeptide made up to two peptide chains A and B (with 21 and 30 amino acids). It activates cyclic AMP (second messenger) which in turn causes the release of calcium ions. Insulin increases the glucose uptake in the peripheral tissues.

8 A False
  B True
  C True
  D False
  E False
Biguanides act by increasing glucose utilization by enhancing anaerobic glycolysis or decreasing gluconeogenesis or by inhibiting intestinal reabsorption of glucose. They have a short half-life of 3 h, but their hypoglycaemic action can be prolonged to between 6 and 14 h. Ketonuria is seen in unstable juvenile diabetics who are treated with insulin and phenformin. Biguanides are not recommended during pregnancy and they are usually prescribed in maturity onset diabetes.

9 A True
  B False
  C True
  D False
  E False
The β-lactamase-resistant penicillins include methicillin, cloxacillin, nafcillin. These drugs are not destroyed by most β-lactamases of staphylococci. These agents are less active against oral cavity anaerobic species than is penicillin G and show no activity against Gram-negative bacilli.

10 Gentamicin
  A Is active against *Klebsiella*
  B Acts by inhibiting the protein biosynthesis of the microsome
  C Can cause a transient rise in alkaline phosphatase
  D Is excreted by glomerular filtration
  E Crosses the blood/brain barrier easily

11 Cephalosporins
  A Cefazolin is easily absorbed from the gastrointestinal tract
  B Cephalexin has a half-life of 40 min
  C Cause eosinopenia
  D Lead to a direct positive Coombs reaction
  E Cephaloridine is nephrotoxic

12 Penicillins
  A Most of the dose of penicillin G is absorbed from the stomach
  B Probenicid blocks renal tubular secretion of penicillin
  C Have an apparent volume of distribution of 50% of total body water
  D 90% of the penicillin in the blood is found in RBCs and 10% in plasma
  E Cross the blood/brain barrier easily

10 A True
   B False
   C True
   D True
   E False

Gentamicin is active against *Klebsiella, Pseudomonas, Escherichia coli* and *Enterocoli*. It acts on the ribosome where it inhibits the protein biosynthesis and decreases the fidelity of translation of the genetic code. Gentamicin is known to cross the blood/brain barrier like penicillins only in infected meninges and is found to cause a rise in alkaline phosphatase and serum transaminases.

11 A False
   B True
   C False
   D True
   E True

Cefazolin is not as well absorbed from the gastrointestinal tract as compared with cephalexin. The cephalosporins cause eosinophilia, urticaria and anaphylaxis as side-effects. In 40% of the patients when large doses of cephalothin are used, a direct positive Coombs reaction is seen. Renal injury due to cephaloridine occurs most often with administration of 6 g or more per day.

12 A False
   B True
   C True
   D False
   E False

After an oral administration, one-third of the dose is absorbed from the intestinal tract and a small portion from the stomach. Some 90% of the penicillins are found in the plasma and 10% in the RBCs. They do not cross intact meninges, but cross the blood/brain barrier in meningitis.

13 Sulphonylureas
A   Stimulate islet cells of pancreas to secrete insulin
B   Are effecctive when given parenterally
C   Tolbutamide reaches its peak concentration in 3–5 h
D   Chlorpropamide is metabolized and excreted via the kidneys
E   Cause pancytopenia

14 Chloramphenicol is used in the treatment of:
A   Typhoid fever
B   Gonorrhoea
C   *Staphylococcus aureus* infections
D   *Haemophilus influenzae*
E   Gas gangrene

15 Antibiotics
A   Aminoglycosides cause misreading of the genetic code
B   Actinomycin D binds to RNA
C   Colchicine inhibits DNA polymerase
D   Chloramphenicol prevents normal association of mRNA with ribosomes
E   Mechlorethamine binds to guanine in base pairs

16 During pregnancy
A   Fibrinolytic activity is reduced
B   Fibrinogen concentration rises from 3.0 g/100 ml to 5.5 g/100 ml
C   Blood volume is decreased at term
D   Excessive blood loss during spontaneous vertex delivery is from episiotomy or trauma to cervix and perineum
E   During delivery, 30% of blood volume can be lost without a change in the haematocrit

13 A True
  B False
  C True
  D False
  E True
Sulphonylureas are effective when given orally. Tolbutamide has a half-life of 5 h. Chlorpropamide is not altered metabolically and is excreted very slowly in unchanged form. Acetohexamide, tolazamide, tolbutamide, chlorpropamide cause leukopenia, agranulocytosis and thrombocytopenia.

14 A True
  B False
  C False
  D True
  E False
Chloramphenicol acts by preventing the addition of new amino acids to the growing peptide chains by interfering with binding of the aminoacyl-tRNA complex with the 50S subunit. It is extremely well absorbed from the gastrointestinal tract, with peak plasma concentrations in about 2 h after ingestion. Chloramphenicol has an extremely broad spectrum of antimicrobial activity, inhibiting aerobic and anaerobic Gram-positive and Gram-negative bacteria, chlamydiae, ricketsiae, mycoplasma. It is bactericidal against *H. influenzae*, *N. meningitidis* and *S. pneumoniae*.

15 A True
  B False
  C True
  D True
  E True
Actinomycin D binds to DNA preventing polymerization of RNA on DNA.

16 A True
  B False
  C False
  D True
  E True
The blood is hypercoagulable and the fibrinogen concentration rises from 3.0 g/l to 5.5 g/l. The blood volume is increased by 40%.

17 Growth hormone secretion
A Is increased during fasting
B Apomorphine decreases it
C Is decreased by non-REM sleep (non-rapid eye movement sleep)
D Is increased by a protein meal
E Is decreased by cortisol

18 Hypocalcaemia is associated with
A Acute pancreatitis
B Cushing's syndrome
C Hypophosphataemia
D Metabolic acidosis
E Papilloedema

19 Primary aldosteronism
A Urinary specific gravity is 1018
B Standard bicarbonate is higher than actual bicarbonate
C Potassium wasting is seen
D Occurs more often in men than women
E Diastolic hypertension is common

20 Drugs and pregnancy
A Teratogenesis may occur if drugs are given between 5 and 12 weeks after the first day of the last menstrual period
B Lithium treatment of the mother can affect skeletal development of the fetus
C Phenolic compounds can cause cataracts in newborns
D Reserpine causes feeding difficulties in a newborn
E Chloroquine can cause fetal renal agenesis

17 A True
B False
C False
D True
E True
Human growth hormone resembles prolactin and human chorionic somatotrophin. Growth hormone (GH) is metabolized rapidly and has a circulating half-life of 6–20 min. The secretion of GH is controlled via the hypothalamus. The factors which increase GH secretion are hypoglycaemia, exercise, fasting, protein meal, glucagon, stressful stimuli, sleep, oestrogens and androgens. The factors which decrease its secretion are REM sleep, glucose, free fatty acids, cortisol.

18 A True
B True
C False
D False
E True
Hyperphosphataemic metabolic alkalosis is associated with hypocalcaemia. Papilloedema occurs with or without raised intracranial pressure.

19 A False
B False
C True
D False
E True
The urinary specific gravity is below 1010 due to the loss of concentrating ability. Actual bicarbonate is higher than standard bicarbonate indicating respiratory acidosis. Aldosteronism is seen commonly in women around 40–50 years of age.

20 A True
B True
C True
D True
E False

21 Adrenal steroids
A Triamcinolone is highly potent in retaining sodium
B Cortisone (25 mg tablet) has twice the anti-inflammatory effect as an equipotent dose of triamcinolone
C Aldosterone is active when swallowed
D Cortisone is converted to hydrocortisone in the liver
E Deoxycortisone is eliminated by first-pass metabolism

22 Thyroid hormones
A Depress mitochondrial respiration
B Increase albumin synthesis
C In excess prolong the reaction time of stretch reflexes
D Cause a fall in peripheral resistance
E Cause a fall in oxygen consumption

23 Calcitonin
A Is secreted by clear cells or C cells
B Normal rate of secretion is about 1.0 mg/day
C Lowers phosphate levels
D Acts by inhibiting the active transport of calcium from bone cells into the extracellular fluid
E Increases renal formation of 1,25-dihydroxycholecalciferol

24 Glucagon
A Is a linear polypeptide
B Is lipogenic
C Has a half-life of 5–10 min
D Its calorigenic action is due to hyperglycaemia
E Secretion is inhibited by glucose

21 A False
    B False
    C False
    D True
    E True

Triamcinolone is an anti-inflammatory and cortisone is only 0.8 times as effective as an anti-inflammatory.

22 A False
    B True
    C False
    D True
    E False

Thyroid hormones stimulate mitochondrial respiration along with phosphorylation and the activity of respiratory enzymes. Thyroid hormones also increase the oxygen consumption.

23 A True
    B False
    C True
    D True
    E False

The normal rate of secretion of calcitonin is 0.5 mg/day and it tends to lower the phosphate and calcium levels.

24 A True
    B False
    C True
    D False
    E True

Glucagon is a lipolytic agent and its calorigenic action is due to increased hepatic deamination of amino acids. Its secretion is inhibited by glucose as opposed to cortisol and exercise which stimulate its secretion.

25 Respiratory changes during pregnancy
   A   Enlarged uterus displaces the diaphragm upwards decreasing the volume of the thoracic cavity
   B   Splinting of the diaphragm occurs in Trendelenburg position
   C   Tidal volume increases by 40% over non-pregnant values
   D   Functional residual capacity remains unaltered
   E   There is a decrease in the lung compliance at term

26 Iodide
   A   Is absorbed from the intestine
   B   Is used in thyroid storm
   C   Potassium iodide 600 mg is given orally every 8 h prior to thyroid surgery
   D   Iodism includes metallic taste, painful salivary glands
   E   Elimination can be enhanced using frusemide

27 During pregnancy:
   A   Haematocrit is low
   B   Plasma volume increases to the maximum at 28 weeks of gestation
   C   Red cell volume does not change much during severe pre-eclampsia
   D   Plasma globulins are increased
   E   There is a considerable fall in phospholipid and non-esterified fatty acids

25 A False
  B True
  C True
  D False
  E False
Although the diaphragm is displaced upward, there is no change in the volume of the thoracic cavity because compensatory increase occurs in transverse and antero-posterior diameter. Functional residual capacity is decreased by up to 18% at term. The lung compliance is unaltered during pregnancy, but increases by 25% following delivery.

26 A True
  B True
  C False
  D True
  E False
Potassium iodide is given 60 mg orally 8 hourly which produces its effect within 1–2 days. A saline diuresis can enhance the elimination of potassium iodide.

27 A True
  B False
  C False
  D True
  E False
The haematocrit during pregnancy is low because of a rise in plasma volume exceeding a rise in red cell volume (down to 34% from 40–42%). Plasma volume increases at 34 weeks of gestation and it is slightly greater in multigravidas and multiple pregnancies. Red cell volume is abnormally low during severe pre-eclampsia. In particular $\alpha1$, $\alpha2$ and β-globulins are increased, while γ-globulins are decreased slightly. There is a considerable rise in phospholipid and non-esterified fatty acids (NEFA). The peripheral utilization of NEFA is increased which results in a high concentration of ketone bodies in blood.

28 Haemodynamic changes during pregnancy
   A   Pressure in inferior vena cava is lowest in the supine position as compared with the lateral position
   B   Circulation time is unaltered in upper parts of the body
   C   Enlargement of the heart is due to deposition of fat
   D   T waves are elevated in lead III in the ECG
   E   During contractions there is a rise in cardiac output

29 During pregnancy:
   A   Arterial PCO_2 falls to 31 mmHg by 16th week of pregnancy
   B   Fall in PCO_2 is due to the influence of progesterone
   C   Respiratory alkalosis of pregnancy facilitates placental transfer of gases
   D   Oxyhaemoglobin dissociation curve is shifted to the right
   E   Closing volume falls by 20% at term

30 Circulatory values in human fetus and newborn
   A   Systolic blood pressure in a newborn is 70 mmHg
   B   Blood flow is high in the pulmonary artery in the fetus
   C   Pulmonary artery pressure is higher in the newborn than in the adults
   D   In the fetus there is a high blood flow through the ductus arteriosus to the aorta
   E   Heart rate is approximately equal in the fetus and newborn

28 A False
B True
C False
D False
E True
The pressure in inferior vena cava in the lateral position is 10–15 mmHg as compared with supine (20–30 mmHg). Circulation time is unaltered in the upper part of the body but slowed in lower limbs. Enlargement of the heart is due to an increase in the thickness of heart muscle and increase in the volume of chambers of the heart. T waves in the ECG are flattened or inverted in lead III due to a left axis deviation. The rise in cardiac output during contractions is due to the expulsion of blood from the uterus into general circulation during contraction.

29 A False
B True
C True
D False
E False
The arterial P_{CO_2} falls to 31 mmHg by the 12th week of pregnancy and it is due to the increased production of progesterone. Oxyhaemoglobin dissociation curve is unchanged. The closing volume is increased in 50% of women at term.

30 A True
B False
C True
D True
E True
There is no blood flow in the pulmonary artery in the fetus, but the systolic pressure is 35/15 mmHg in the newborn as compared with 30/10 mmHg in adults.

31 Hypercalcaemia
A Is seen in sarcoidosis
B Occurs in acromegaly
C Causes diarrhoea
D Is associated with band keratopathy
E Causes metabolic alkalosis

32 During pregnancy
A By the third month the heart rate of the mother increases to 85 bpm
B Diastolic blood pressure falls slightly in mid-pregnancy
C Supine hypotension occurs in 20% of women when they lie supine for 5 minutes
D Systolic blood pressure is highest in the sitting position
E During second stage of labour, systolic blood pressure rises by 30 mmHg

33 Spironolactone
A Is a steroid
B Decreases calcium excretion
C Dose is 100 mg administered IV
D Induces hyperkalaemia
E Causes an increased excretion of water and electrolytes

34 Insulin
A Synalbumin has anti-insulin activity
B Half-life of insulin is 45 min
C Insulin binds to RBCs and brain tissue
D 80% of the secreted insulin is degraded in the liver and kidneys
E Enzyme capable of dissipating the disulphide linkages is hepatic glutathione insulin transhydrogenase

31 A True
    B True
    C False
    D True
    E False
Hypercalcaemia is associated with anorexia, vomiting and constipation. The blood gas analysis shows hyperchloraemic metabolic acidosis. Band keratopathy consists of grey or white granular bands in the cornea.

32 A False
    B True
    C False
    D True
    E True
The heart rate in a pregnant woman is around 78 bpm at the third month, which increases to 85 bpm in late pregnancy. Supine hypotension occurs in 10% of women when they lie supine for 5 min.

33 A True
    B False
    C False
    D True
    E True
Spironolactone is used in the treatment of refractory oedema and it is given 100 mg orally in divided doses. When used in conjunction with thiazides it induces hyperkalaemia. It increases calcium excretion through a direct effect on the tubular transport.

34 A True
    B False
    C False
    D True
    E True
Insulin has a half-life of 10–20 min and is fixed to many tissues, except RBCs and brain tissue. Hepatic glutathione insulin transhydrogenase breaks the insulin molecule into A and B chains.

35 Glucocorticoids
A Exert anti-insulin action
B Inhibit ACTH secretion
C Help in restoring the muscle to normal following fatigue
D Decrease PR interval in ECG when they are in excess
E Deficiency causes inability to concentrate

36 Glucocorticoids
A Are bound to an albumin called transcortin
B Half-life of cortisol is 50 min
C Transcortin levels are decreased during pregnancy
D Cortisol is reduced to tetrahydrocortisol
E Cortisone is secreted by the adrenal gland

37 Fetal respiration and circulation at birth
A Fetal haemoglobin binds effectively to 2,3-DPG
B At birth expansion of the lungs occurs due to a markedly negative intrapleural pressure
C After the lungs expand, the pulmonary vascular resistance falls
D Prostaglandins prevent the closure of the ductus arteriosus before birth
E At birth, the peripheral resistance in the fetus falls

35 A True
   B True
   C True
   D True
   E True
Glucocorticoids make diabetes worse by exerting ant-insulin action. ACTH is increased in adrenalectomized animals. In patients with adrenal insufficiency the personality changes seen are irritability, apprehension and inability to concentrate.

36 A False
   B False
   C False
   D True
   E False
Glucocorticoids are bound to an α-globulin called transcortin or corticosteroid-binding globulin (CBG). The half-life of cortisol is between 60 and 90 min and that of corticosterone is 50 min. Transcortin levels are increased during pregnancy and decreased in patients with cirrhosis, nephrosis and multiple myeloma. Cortisol is reduced to tetrahydrocortisol which is then conjugated to glucuronic acid. Cortisone is synthesized in the liver and not in the adrenal gland.

37 A False
   B True
   C True
   D True
   E False
Fetal haemoglobin binds less effectively than adult haemoglobin to 2,3-DPG. At birth the expansion of lungs occurs due to intrapleural pressures of -30 to -50 mmHg. After the lungs expand the pulmonary vascular resistance falls to less than 20% of the value *in utero*.

38 Prostaglandins (PG)
A   Are a series of closely related 20-carbon saturated fatty acids
B   Are inactivated in the renal cortex
C   Have a long half-life
D   Play a role in the transfer of RBCs through the capillaries
E   Prostaglandin A lowers blood pressure

39 Insulin secretion
A   Is stimulated by leucine
B   Is inhibited by theophylline
C   Somatostatin has no effect
D   Is increased by galactose
E   Is blocked by atropine

40 Insulin facilitates glucose uptake in:
A   Intestinal mucosa
B   Fibroblasts
C   Crystalline lens of the eye
D   Pituitary
E   Red blood cells

38 A False
    B True
    C False
    D True
    E True

Prostaglandins are 20-carbon unsaturated fatty acids containing a cyclopentane ring. They have short half-lives and are metabolized to inactive compounds by oxidation and isomerization in the renal cortex, the lungs and liver. Prostaglandins regulate the capacity of RBCs to undergo deformation in passing through capillaries.

39 A True
    B False
    C False
    D False
    E True

Theophylline stimulates insulin secretion as compared with somatostatin which inhibits it. Galactose has no effect, although the entry of glucose, xylose and arabinose into cells is facilitated by insulin.

40 A False
    B True
    C True
    D True
    E False

Insulin is an active acidic protein with a molecular weight of 5600. It is composed of two polypeptides, called A and B chains which are covalently joined by two interchain disulphide bonds. Insulin stimulates the transport of glucose into muscle and fat cells. It is involved in the interaction with a cell-surface receptor.

41 Calcium
- A Normal calcium levels are 8.5–10.5 mg/100 ml
- B About 2 mg of plasma calcium/100 ml is ultrafiltrable calcium
- C Hypocalcaemia is seen in chronic renal failure
- D Hypercalcaemia leads to marked lassitude
- E Calcium is lost daily in the skin and sweat

42 Insulin
- A Decreases protein synthesis in ribosomes
- B Increases cyclic AMP levels in the liver
- C Increases ketone uptake in the muscle
- D Activates hormone-sensitive lipase
- E Increases potassium uptake

41 A True
    B False
    C True
    D True
    E True
About 5 mg/100 ml of plasma calcium is ultrafiltrable calcium.
Hypercalcaemia leads to marked lassitude, muscular weakness and
thirst.

42 A False
    B False
    C True
    D False
    E True
Insulin increases the protein synthesis in ribosomes and decreases
cyclic AMP levels in the liver. It also inhibits hormone-sensitive
lipase.

5 Gastrointestinal system

1 **Ranitidine**
   A When injected IV has a half-life of 1 h
   B Bioavailability is 50–60%
   C Does not impair hepatic elimination of drugs
   D Has no influence on gastroduodenal reflux
   E Is bound to plasma proteins

2 **Metoclopramide**
   A Diminishes the sensitivity of visceral nerves to local emetics
   B Decreases the tone of lower oesophageal sphincter
   C Central effects can be antagonized by atropine
   D Can cause drowsiness
   E Acts on the chemoreceptor trigger zone

3 **Cimetidine**
   A Is effective in Zollinger–Ellison syndrome
   B Can cause a rise in acid phosphatase
   C Has a half-life of 4 h
   D Is metabolized and excreted totally via the kidneys
   E Can cause gynaecomastia

Gastrointestinal system: Answers

1 A False
   B True
   C True
   D False
   E True

The reduction in gastric acid output is associated with a long-lasting increase in pH. Ranitidine is 15% bound to plasma proteins and has a volume of distribution between 1.2 and 1.8 l/kg.

2 A True
   B False
   C False
   D True
   E True

Metoclopramide is a chlorinated procainamide derivative. It acts by antagonizing the peripheral dopaminergic (D_2-) receptors, augmenting the peripheral cholinergic action and by a direct action on smooth muscle. Metoclopramide raises the threshold for vomiting at the chemoreceptor trigger zone. It increases the tone of the lower oesophageal sphincter, accelerating gastric emptying. Metoclopramide causes a transient rise in aldosterone secretion and stimulates prolactin release. It can be administered orally, IV or IM. The adult dose is 10 mg 8 hourly by all routes.

3 A True
   B False
   C False
   D False
   E True

Cimetidine has a half-life of 2 h and is largely excreted unchanged via the kidneys (70%). It causes a rise in alkaline phosphatase.

4 Cimetidine
  A Has a half-life of 2 h
  B Can cause sexual dysfunction in males
  C Causes a fall in plasma creatinine
  D Interacts with anticoagulants and increases prothrombin time by 35%
  E Hastens gastric emptying

5 Antacids
  A Magnesium trisilicate reacts quickly to form magnesium chloride
  B Calcium carbonate does not cause any acid/base imbalance
  C Aluminium hydroxide binds phosphate in the gut and is not absorbed
  D Calcium chloride causes diarrhoea
  E Magnesium carbonate is highly effective

6 H₂ receptor blockers
  A Ranitidine binds to androgen receptors
  B Cimetidine binds to cytochrome P-450
  C Cimetidine causes thrombocytosis
  D Ranitidine inhibits the metabolism of warfarin
  E Ranitidine causes reversible confusion

7 Gastric juice
  A The volume secreted by a man in 24 h is 2000–2500 ml
  B Fasting gastric juice has a pH between 0.9 and 1.2
  C Chloride ions of the hydrochloric acid are secreted by a passive mechanism
  D In highly acidic gastric juice, sodium and potassium chlorides are present in small amounts
  E Sodium and hydrogen ions play an important role in the regulation of intragastric hydrogen ion concentration

4 A True
  B True
  C False
  D False
  E False
Cimetidine is an imidazole derivative. It acts by inhibiting all phases of gastric acid secretion. After a rapid IV injection, bradycardias and dysrhythmias may occur. Cimetidine has a weak antiandrogenic effect which can lead to gynaecomastia. It is used in the treatment of peptic ulcer, reflux oesophagitis and Zollinger–Ellison syndrome. The normal adult dose is 400 mg 12 hourly or 800 mg as a single nocturnal dose. The adult IV dose is up to 2.4 g/day.

5 A False
  B True
  C True
  D False
  E False
Magnesium trisilicate reacts slowly to form magnesium chloride. Calcium chloride causes constipation and magnesium carbonate is least effective.

6 A False
  B True
  C False
  D False
  E True
Cimetidine and not ranitidine causes gynaecomastia and occasionally impotence. The former retards the oxidative phase of hepatic drug metabolism by binding to microsomal cytochrome P-450. Again, cimetidine, and not ranitidine, blocks the metabolism of warfarin, phenytoin and aminophylline. Both the H_2 blockers cause reversible confusion.

7 A True
  B True
  C False
  D True
  E True
The cells of gastric glands secrete about 2500 ml of gastric juice daily. It contains cations (Na^+, K^+, Mg^{2+}, H^+), anions (Cl^-, HPO_4^{2-}, SO_4^{2-}), pepsins I–III etc. The glands secrete HCl and the gastric muscosa secretes bicarbonate.

8 Cyclic 3'5'-adenosine monophosphate (cyclic AMP)
  A   Is derived from adenosine monophosphate
  B   Adenylate cyclase is located in the cell membrane
  C   Glucagon causes lipolysis by decreasing intracellular cyclic AMP
  D   Prostaglandins antagonize the effects of agents that stimulate cyclic AMP
  E   Urinary cyclic AMP is decreased in patients with hypoparathyroidism

9 Pancreatic juice
  A   Is hyperosmotic compared with the plasma
  B   Calcium concentration is higher than in plasma
  C   Pancreatic amylase is secreted in an active form
  D   Chymotrypsin digests casein
  E   Protein content ranges from 0.1 to 0.3%

10 Vitamins
  A   Pantothenic acid is a constituent of CoA
  B   A deficiency of thiamine causes glossitis and cheilosis
  C   Niacin is a constituent of NAD^+ and $NADP^+$
  D   Vitamin E is necessary for hydroxylation of lysine
  E   Vitamin K is present in leafy green vegetables

8 A False
  B True
  C False
  D True
  E False
Cyclic AMP is derived from ATP in the presence of an enzyme adenylate cyclase. Glucagon causes lipolysis by increasing intracellular cyclic AMP. An increase in cyclic AMP is produced by parathyroid hormone. Urinary cyclic AMP excretion is decreased in patients with pseudohypoparathyroidism.

9 A False
  B False
  C True
  D True
  E True
Pancreatic juice is iso-osmotic with plasma and has a lower calcium level than plasma ($1.7 + 0.3$ mmol/kg of H_2O).

10 A True
  B False
  C True
  D False
  E True
The source of pantothenic acid is eggs, liver and yeast. Its deficiency causes dermatitis, enteritis and adrenal insufficiency. A deficiency of thiamine (vitamin B1) causes beri beri and neuritis, whereas a deficiency of riboflavin (vitamin B2) causes glossitis and cheilosis. Vitamin C is necessary for the hydroxylation of lysine in collagen synthesis, whereas vitamin E acts as an antioxidant.

11 Protein metabolism
A Protein provides 20% of the energy requirements
B Animal proteins are first-class proteins
C Human pepsin causes coagulation of milk
D Amino acids are absorbed in the pylorus of the stomach
E Trypsin digests protein to long-chain peptides

12 Lipids
A Cerebrosides contain galactose and fatty acids
B Triglycerides are esters of glycerol and two fatty acids
C Oleic acid is an unsaturated fatty acid
D Sphingomyelins contain cholesterol and its derivatives
E Palmitic acid is a saturated fatty acid

13 Carbohydrate metabolism
A Glucose-6-phosphatase enzyme facilitates conversion of glucose to glucose 6-phosphate
B During aerobic glycolysis, ATP production is 19 times greater than anaerobic conditions
C For 1 mol of blood glucose metabolized aerobically in the Embden–Meyerhof pathway, 36 mol of ATP are generated
D Amount of ATP generated depends upon the amount of NADH converted
E Phosphorylase converts glycogen to glucose 1-phosphate

11 A False
   B True
   C True
   D False
   E False
Proteins provide 5–10% of the energy requirements, the energy value being 17 kJ/g. Except gelatin, all animal proteins are first-class proteins. The human pepsin causes coagulation of milk because of its renin-like activity. Amino acids from food protein and endogenous sources are readily absorbed from the small intestine.

12 A True
   B False
   C True
   D False
   E True
Triglycerides are esters of glycerol and three fatty acids. Sphingomyelins contain esters of fatty acid, phosphate, choline and amino alcohol with sphingosine.

13 A False
   B True
   C False
   D False
   E True
Hexokinase takes part in the conversion of glucose to glucos-6-phosphate, whereas glucose-6-phosphatase facilitates conversion of glucose 6-phosphate to glucose. For 1 mol of glucose metabolized aerobically, there are 38 mol of ATP generated. The amount of ATP generated depends upon the amount of NADPH converted to NADH and then oxidized.

14 Lipid metabolism
A Fat in the diet carries fat-soluble vitamins A, C, K
B About 25% of neutral fat is hydrolysed in the upper small intestine
C Short-chain fatty acids form water-soluble micelles
D Bile salts are essential for the absorption of fat
E Normal daily diet in the UK contains 40–80 g of neutral fat

15 Essential amino acids
A Valine
B Isoleucine
C Tyrosine
D Lysine
E Serine

16 DNA and RNA
A DNA is present in the nucleus
B RNA carries a genetic message
C Formation of tRNA (transfer RNA) is catalysed by the enzyme RNA polymerase
D Molecules of tRNA contain 70–80 nitrogenous bases
E DNA passes from one generation to the next in germs cells

14 A False
    B True
    C False
    D True
    E True
Fat in the diet carries fat-soluble vitamins such as A, D, K. Most short-chain fatty acids are absorbed directly, the long-chain fatty acids and monoglycerides, in combination with bile salts, form water-soluble micelles.

15 A True
    B True
    C False
    D True
    E False
The essential amino acids are valine, leucine, isoleucine, threonine, methionine, phenylalanine, tryptophan and lysine.

16 A True
    B False
    C False
    D True
    E True
DNA is present in the nucleus and the mitochondria and is made up of two long nucleotide chains containing adenine, guanine, thymine and cytosine. It carries a genetic message which is coded by the sequence of purine and pyrimidine bases in the nucleotide chains. The message is transferred to the sites of protein synthesis in the cytoplasm by RNA. Strands of DNA serve as templates by lining up complementary bases for the formation in the nucleus of messenger RNA (mRNA) and soluble or transfer RNA (tRNA).

6 Renal and hepatic system

1 **Thiazides**
   A Produce dose-dependent sodium diuresis
   B Chlorthiazide is lipid soluble
   C Causes hypokalaemic acidosis
   D Can decrease the blood pressure by 10% on its own
   E Arteriolar dilatation is due to ion shift in the vessel wall

2 **Frusemide**
   A Its action lasts for 4 h
   B Can lower serum calcium in hypercalcaemia
   C Acts exclusively by venodilatation
   D Is a sulphonamide derivative
   E Acts on the distal tubule

3 **Allopurinol**
   A Inhibits the terminal steps in uric acid synthesis
   B Facilitates the action of xanthine oxidase
   C Is a uricosuric agent
   D Has a half-life of 2–3 h
   E Is effective in polycythaemia vera

Renal and hepatic system: Answers

1 A True
   B False
   C False
   D True
   E True
The main site of action of thiazides is the early distal tubule.
Chlorthiazide inhibits bicarbonate transport in the proximal tubule.
Chlorthiazide potentiates the antihypertensive action of ganglion
blockers. The renal effects of thiazides depends on the physiological
water and electrolyte balance, functional status of the cardiovascular
system and kidney.

2 A True
   B True
   C False
   D True
   E False
Frusemide is a sulphonamide (anthralenic) derivative. It acts by
inhibiting active chloride ion reabsorption in the proximal tubule
and ascending limb of the loop of Henle. The action at cellular level
is exerted by inhibition of Na^+/K^+-ATPase. It is used in the
treatment of oedema of renal, cardiac and hepatic origin.

3 A True
   B False
   C True
   D True
   E True
Allopurinol is a xanthine oxidase inhibitor which increases the renal
excretion of urate. It is effective in treating hyperuricaemia seen in
polycythaemia vera.

4 Diuretics
A Frusemide inhibits the chloride reabsorption in distal tubules
B Triamterene inhibits Na^+/K^+ exchange in the distal tubules by acting directly
C Acetazolamide decreases hydrogen secretion
D Xanthines decrease the glomerular filtration rate
E Ethyl alcohol inhibits vasopressin secretion

5 Ethacrynic acid
A Is related to frusemide
B Inhibits absorption of chloride in the loop of Henle
C Increases the excretion of potassium and hydrogen ion
D Its maximum activity occurs in 6 h
E Can cause deafness

6 Amiodarone
A Is administered twice a day
B Causes corneal deposition
C Contains iodine
D Is the treatment of choice in heart failure
E Causes peripheral neuropathy

7 Thiazides
A Act on the proximal convoluted tubules
B Cause hyperchloraemic alkalosis
C Can cause thrombocytopenia
D Have an onset of action in 2 h
E Increase the peripheral resistance

4 A False
   B True
   C True
   D False
   E True
Frusemide acts on the loop of Henle. Unlike spironolactone (another potassium-sparing diuretic), triamterene inhibits Na^+/K^+ exchange in the distal tubule by inhibiting the action of aldosterone. Acetazolamide decreases hydrogen secretion, thus resulting in an increase in Na^+ and K^+ excretion. Theophylline and caffeine decrease tubular reabsorption of sodium and increase GFR.

5 A False
   B True
   C True
   D False
   E True
Ethacrynic acid is a synthetic drug whose maximum activity is reached in 2 hours and diuresis persists for 6–8 h

6 A False
   B True
   C True
   D False
   E True
Amiodarone, because of its very long half-life, is given once a day. Iodine present in it when released can cause disorders of thyroid function. It is used in the treatment of supraventricular tachycardias, ventricular tachycardia, atrial fibrillation and flutter. The side-effects include peripheral neuropathy, diffuse pulmonary alveolitis and hepatic damage.

7 A False
   B False
   C True
   D True
   E False
Thiazides act on the distal convoluted tubules with a duration of action of 12–24 h. It decreases peripheral resistance and causes hypochloraemic alkalosis associated with hypokalaemia.

8 Bendrofluazide
A   Causes decreased urinary excretion of sodium
B   Decreases plasma volume
C   Causes an increase in the cardiac output
D   Enhances gluconeogenesis, thus increasing the blood sugar concentration
E   Can cause hypercalcaemia

9 Proximal renal tubular acidosis
A   Occurs following rejection of a renal transplant
B   85–90% of bicarbonate ions that are filtered by glomeruli are absorbed
C   Hypophosphataemia occurs
D   Urine has a high pH
E   Pseudofractures can be seen

10 Vasopressin
A   Secretion increases when lying recumbent
B   Is increased in haemorrhage
C   Is increased in the presence of hypotonic plasma
D   Acts by increasing intracellular cyclic AMP
E   Decreases blood flow in the renal medulla

8 A False
   B True
   C False
   D False
   E True
Bendrofluazide is a thiazide which acts by inhibiting sodium ion reabsorption resulting in an increased urinary excretion of sodium, potassium and water. It exerts its antihypertensive effect by decreasing the plasma volume and systemic vascular resistance. It also causes a slight decrease in the cardiac output. Bendrofluazide decreases the renal blood flow and may also cause a reduction in the glomerular filtration rate. It increases the blood sugar concentration by enhancing glycogenolysis and insulin secretion. Bendrofluazide can cause hypokalaemia and hypercalcaemia, which may precipitate digoxin toxicity.

9 A True
   B True
   C True
   D False
   E False
Both proximal and distal renal tubular acidosis are seen in patients following rejection of a renal transplant. The urinary pH is normal when the metabolic acidosis is severe because the reabsorption of bicarbonate ions is completed in the proximal tubules. Pseudofractures are seen in patients with distal renal tubular acidosis.

10 A False
    B True
    C True
    D True
    E True
Vasopressin is secreted by the posterior pituitary gland. Along with oxytocin it is a neural hormone. Vasopressin (also called ADH) causes retention of the water by the kidney. It increases the blood pressure by an action on the smooth muscle of the arterioles. There are two types of vasopressin receptors. V_1 receptors are present in blood vessels, brain and glomerular mesangial cells and they mediate the vasoconstrictor action. V_2 receptors are found in the thick ascending limb of the loop of Henle and the collecting duct and they mediate the antidiuretic effect. Vasopressin is rapidly inactivated in the liver and the kidney. It has a half-life of 18 minutes.

11 Potassium and urine formation
   A   Potassium is actively reabsorbed in the distal tubular cells
   B   Potassium excretion is decreased when the amount of sodium reaching the distal tubules is low
   C   When the hydrogen ion secretion is increased, excretion of potassium is increased
   D   In hypokalaemia the urine is alkaline
   E   Aldosterone increases the secretion of potassium

12 Renal circulation
   A   In a resting adult the kidneys receive 1.2 l of blood/min
   B   Renal plasma flow is measured using *para*-aminohippuric acid (PAH) infusion
   C   Blood flow to the renal medulla is higher than to the renal cortex
   D   Hypoxia causes renal vasodilatation
   E   Prostaglandins increase the blood flow in the renal medulla

13 Glomerular filtration rate (GFR)
   A   A substance suitable for measuring GFR should be absorbed or secreted by tubules
   B   Substances with a molecular weight above 60 000 are easily filtered
   C   The filtration fraction is between 0.16 and 0.20 in normal subjects
   D   Ureteral obstruction increases GFR
   E   Efferent arteriolar constriction decreases GFR

11 A False
  B True
  C False
  D False
  E True
Potassium is actively absorbed in the proximal tubules and t!.en secreted into the fluid by the distal tubular cells. The potassium excretion is decreased when the hydrogen ion secretion is increased. In hypokalaemia all the potassium is reabsorbed in the distal tubules and in exchange hydrogen ion is excreted, thus producing acidic urine. Aldosterone increases the secretion of potassium and hydrogen and also the tubular reabsorption of sodium.

12 A True
  B True
  C False
  D False
  E False
The adult kidneys at rest receive just under 25% of the cardiac output. PAH is a substance which is filtered by the glomeruli and secreted by tubules. Renal plasma flow is measured as amount of PAH in the urine/amount of PAH in the plasma. The blood flow to the renal cortex is about 4–5 ml/g of kidney tissue per minute as compared with 1–2 ml/g in the outer medulla. Hypoxia causes vasoconstriction, and prostaglandins increase the blood flow in the renal cortex but decrease it in the medulla.

13 A False
  B False
  C True
  D False
  E False
A substance suitable for GFR should not be reabsorbed or secreted by tubules, freely filtered and non-protein bound. Substances that are filtered in large amounts have molecular weights less than 60 000, but diameter rather than molecular weight determines whether a given molecule will be filtered. Filtration fraction is the ratio of GFR to the renal plasma flow. GFR is maintained when efferent arteriolar constriction is greater than afferent arteriolar constriction.

14 Aldosterone
  A Has a half-life of 40 min
  B Is converted in the kidneys and liver to 18-glucuronide
  C Acts on the epithelium of the loop of Henle and collecting duct
  D Increases the potassium level in the muscles and brain cells
  E Produces a potassium diuresis leading to alkaline urine

15 Anatomy of the nephron
  A Proximal convoluted tubule is 15 mm long
  B Nephrons with glomeruli in the outer portions of the renal cortex have long loops of Henle
  C The walls of afferent arteriole adjacent to the thick ascending limb of the loop of Henle contain the juxtaglomerular cells
  D Macula densa is the point where the loop of Henle ends
  E The total length of nephrons, including the collecting ducts, is less than 100 mm

16 Urinary concentration
  A Destruction of renal lymphatics increases renal concentrating ability
  B Hypokalaemia causes polyuria
  C The urine is concentrated in dehydrated patients
  D Sodium chloride in large doses causes osmotic diuresis
  E Concentration of urine in people receiving osmotic diuretics is equal to that of plasma

14 A False
    B True
    C False
    D True
    E False
Aldosterone acts on the distal tubule and the collecting duct and has a half-life of 20 min. It produces a potassium diuresis leading to acidic urine.

15 A True
    B False
    C True
    D True
    E True
The proximal convoluted tubule is 15 mm long and 55 μm in diameter. Nephrons in the outer portion of the renal cortex have short loops of Henle as compared with those with glomeruli in the juxtamedullary regions of the cortex which have long loops. The juxtaglomerular cells (which secrete renin), macula densa and few granulated cells are collectively called the juxtaglomerular apparatus. The total length of nephrons, including the collecting ducts, is between 45 and 65 mm.

16 A False
    B True
    C True
    D True
    E True
Destruction of renal lymphatics decreases the concentrating ability of the kidneys because it permits proteins to accumulate, thus reducing the osmotic gradient along which reabsorbed water moves into vasa recta.

17 Tubular function
A   Glucose is removed by passive transport
B   The transfer maximum of glucose (Tm) is 375 mg/min for men
C   Amino acids are removed by active transport
D   Sodium is actively transported out of the tubular fluid in the collecting ducts
E   The lumen of the loop of Henle is positively charged as compared with the extracellular fluid

18 Water excretion
A   Approximately 70% of the water filtered is reabsorbed
B   The tubular fluid in the proximal tubule is isotonic
C   Ascending limb of loop of Henle is permeable to water
D   About 5% of the water is reabsorbed in the loop of Henle
E   Vasopressin decreases the permeability of epithelium of collecting ducts to water

19 Serum osmolality
A   A high serum osmolality is seen in salicylate poisoning
B   Normal urine/serum osmolality ratio is less than 1
C   Is low in dumping syndrome
D   A normal corrected serum osmolality (260–280 mOsm/kg) indicates that the sodium concentration of extracellular fluid is normal
E   The normal range of osmolality is 275–290 mOsm/kg of serum

17 A False
    B True
    C True
    D True
    E False

Glucose is removed by active transport. The amount of glucose reabsorbed is proportionate to the amount filtered and thus to the plasma glucose level up to the tubular maximum of glucose (Tm), but when the TmG exceeds this, the amount of glucose in the urine rises.

18 A False
    B True
    C False
    D True
    E False

Approximately 88% of the water filtered is reabsorbed. As water moves passively out of the tubule along the osmotic gradients it becomes isotonic in the proximal tubules. The descending limb of the loop of Henle is permeable and the ascending loop impermeable to water. Some 75% of the water is absorbed in the proximal tubules, 15% in the distal tubules and 4.8% in collecting ducts. Vasopressin increases the permeability of the epithelium of collecting ducts to water.

19 A True
    B False
    C False
    D True
    E True

Osmolarity is defined as a molar solution containing 1 g molecular weight of a substance dissolved in a solvent to make 1 litre. Osmolality is defined as a molal solution which contains 1 g molecular weight of a substance dissolved in 1000 g of a solvent. It is determined by measuring the depression of the freezing point of a solution, compared with water using an osmometer. A high serum osmolality is seen in salicylate poisoning, liver failure, alcohol overdose and diabetes. The normal urine/serum osmolality ratio is between 1 and 5. It is low in diabetes insipidus due to water deprivation. The normal serum osmolality in males is between 275 and 290 and in women the values are 5–10 mOsm/kg less than men.

20 Magnesium
  A Hypomagnesaemia occurs with frusemide therapy
  B Magnesium loss occurs in diabetic ketoacidosis
  C Low magnesium levels cause prolonged P-R interval
  D High levels of magnesium cause hypotension
  E Commonest cause of hypermagnesaemia is renal failure

21 Acute renal failure
  A Serum sodium and chloride are low
  B Serum bicarbonate increases with a fall in pH
  C Can occur in patients with cirrhosis of the liver
  D Blood urea nitrogen is increased
  E There is low urinary urea and creatinine

22 Water loss
  A Thirst is the earliest symptom
  B Haematocrit falls
  C Sodium falls
  D Specific gravity of the urine increases
  E Skin of the patient may have a 'rubbery' feeling

20 A False
B True
C False
D True
E True

Hypomagnesaemia is seen following treatment with organic mercurials or thiazides. High levels of magnesium cause prolonged P-R interval, whereas low levels lead to premature atrial or ventricular contractions. Hypotension is due to peripheral vasodilatation in patients with hypermagnesaemia.

21 A True
B False
C True
D True
E False

In acute renal failure there is a fall in serum bicarbonate and pH. Hepatorenal syndrome is seen due to glomerulotubular imbalance caused by toxins.

22 A True
B False
C False
D True
E True

Thirst occurs when the water loss is about 2% of the body weight. Haematocrit rises above 50% and hypernatraemia (> 145 meq/l) indicates that there is too little water for the sodium and other solutes in the body. Skin turgor remains normal as compared with sodium loss where it is lost.

7 Haemopoietic system

1 Heparin
A Is a strongly alkaline mucopolysaccharide
B Action lasts for 6 h
C Prothrombin time is the laboratory test used to control the dose
D After IV injection, 50% of the heparin is dissipated
E Heparin is also called 'clearing factor'

2 Haemoglobin
A Globin moiety consists of six polypeptide chains
B Haemoglobin A has its ferrous ion oxidized to the ferric form by the nitrites
C Consists of α- and β-chains
D Methaemoglobin can carry oxygen
E Dissolved oxygen obeys Henry's law

3 Myoglobin
A Is an iron-containing pigment
B Binds to 4 mol of oxygen/mol
C Has a dissociation curve with a rectangular hyperbola shape
D Releases oxygen only at low PO_2
E Takes up oxygen from haemoglobin in the blood

Haemopoietic system: Answers

1   A   False
    B   False
    C   False
    D   True
    E   True

Heparin is a strongly acidic mucopolysaccharide whose action lasts for 4 h. Partial thromboplastin time is a specific laboratory test used to control the dose. Heparin clears plasma which is turbid due to the presence of chylomicrons.

2   A   False
    B   True
    C   True
    D   False
    E   True

Haemoglobin is a protein with a molecular weight of 64 450. It is made up of 4 subunits. Each subunit contains a haem moiety combined to a polypeptide. Haem is an iron-containing porphyrin derivative; the globin portion makes up the polypeptides.

3   A   True
    B   False
    C   True
    D   True
    E   True

Myoglobin, an iron-containing pigment, binds to 1 mol of oxygen. As opposed to haemoglobin (with a sigmoid-shaped curve), myoglobin has dissociation curve that is a rectangular hyperbola shape.

4 Lymphocytes

  A Precursor of T-lymphocyte originates in bone marrow
  B T-cells are responsible for rejection of allogenic grafts
  C B-cells have a surface marker for IgA
  D Surface IgG and IgM recognize antigens
  E Interferon is released in the presence of phytohaemagglutinin

5 Viscosity of blood

  A Is increased in burns
  B Deoxygenated blood in sickle cell disease decreases it
  C Is increased in hypovolaemia
  D Deformed cell causes a rise
  E Vessel diameter has no effect

6 Clotting tests

  A Coagulation time varies between 5 and 7 min
  B Quick prothrombin time varies between 14 and 16 s
  C Clot retracts within a couple of hours in patients with thrombocytopenia
  D Normal bleeding time is 150 s
  E Partial thromboplastin time depends on the presence of Factors VIII and IX

7 Blood coagulation

  A Fibrinogen is present in low concentrations in patients with liver disease
  B Calcium ions are required to convert fibrin monomer to fibrin threads
  C Heparin is secreted by circulating eosinophil cells which are similar to mast cells
  D Haemophiliacs have a lack of Factor VIII and IX
  E Normal prothrombin time is between 20 and 30 s

4 A   True
    B   True
    C   False
    D   True
    E   True
Lymphocytes are formed in the bone marrow, lymph nodes, thymus and spleen in the adult. They are the key constituents of the immune system. There are two classes of lymphocytes. T-lymphocytes and B-lymphocytes. The T-lymphocytes (thymus-dependent lymphocytes) are concerned with cellular immunity. B-lymphocytes are concerned with cellular immunity.

5 A   True
    B   False
    C   True
    D   False
    E   True
RBC aggregation is increased in patients with burns due to alteration in the plasma proteins.

6 A   False
    B   True
    C   False
    D   True
    E   True
The normal coagulation time is between 9 and 11 min. Clot retraction is abnormal in patients with thrombocytopenia but normal in haemophiliacs.

7 A   True
    B   True
    C   False
    D   True
    E   False
Heparin is secreted by the circulating basophils which are similar to the mast cells. The normal prothrombin time is about 12 s.

8 Plasma proteins
   A γ-globulin is increased in multiple myeloma
   B   Injury and chronic infection cause a fall in fibrinogen
   C   Ceruloplasmin is increased in Wilson's disease
   D   Transferrin transports iron from the gastrointestinal tract to the bone marrow
   E   Haptoglobins show racial differences

9 Haemoglobinopathies
   A   In sickle cell anaemia, haemoglobin S molecules, when deoxygenated, form tactoids
   B   In haemoglobin S, glutamic acid is substituted for valine in the sixth of 146 amino acids
   C   Anisocytosis and target cells are seen in patients with thalassaemia
   D   In haemoglobin C disease, lysine replaces glutamic acid in position 4 of the β-chain position
   E   In long-standing sickle cell disease, renal dysfunction occurs

10 Lymph
   A   Contains all the coagulation factors
   B   An increase in capillary pressure increases lymph flow
   C   Hypoxia decreases the lymph flow
   D   10% dextrose increases the lymph flow
   E   Muscle movement does not affect the lymph flow

8 A True
  B False
  C False
  D True
  E True
There is no change in fibrinogen level in patients with infection or acute injury. Wilson's disease (also called hepatolenticular degeneration) is a familial disorder of copper metabolism in which the plasma copper-binding protein ceruloplasmin is low.

9 A True
  B False
  C True
  D False
  E True
In haemoglobin S, valine is substituted for glutamic acid in the sixth of 146 amino acids. In haemoglobin C disease lysine replaces glutamic acid in the sixth position of the β-chain.

10 A True
  B True
  C False
  D True
  E False
Lymph has the same concentration of chloride ions as plasma (101 mmol/l) and interstitial fluid (116 mmol/l) and a lower concentration of protein (lymph 26 g/l) than plasma (71 g/l) and slightly higher than interstitial fluid (1 g/l).

11   Clotting factors
   A   Factor IX is also called Stuart–Prower factor
   B   Factor V is a labile factor
   C   Hageman Factor is also called Contact Factor
   D   Fibrin-stabilizing factor is Factor VIII
   E   Thrombin is required to convert proaccelerin

12   Plasma proteins
   A   Molecular weight of albumin is 69 000
   B   High-density lipoproteins facilitate lipid transport
   C   Ceruloplasmin helps in iron transport
   D   Plasma concentration of fibrinogen is 4 g/l
   E   About 30% of albumin is replaced daily

13   Red blood cells (RBC)
   A   Are biconcave with a mean diameter of 5 μm
   B   Contain 34 g of haemoglobin/100 ml of cells
   C   Haemocytoblasts are their precursors
   D   Erythropoietin functions effectively in patients with renal failure
   E   Lack of vitamin B12 inhibits red cell production

14   Plasma proteins
   A   Molecular weight of normal plasma albumin is 50 000
   B   Albumin has a half-life of 15 days
   C   Molecular weight of globulins is 150 000
   D α-globulins carry lipids
   E   Most antibodies are γ-globulins

11 A False
  B True
  C True
  D True
  E True

The coagulation factors are divided into three groups: the vitamin K-dependent group which consists of Factors II, VII, IX, X which are synthesized in the liver; the fibrinogen group which consists of Factors I, V, VIII, XIII which are consumed during coagulation; the contact group which is made up of Factors XI and XII. They are involved in the initiation of coagulation by contact with a foreign surface.

12 A True
  B True
  C False
  D True
  E False

Plasma protein consists of albumin, globulin and fibrinogen. The globulin fraction is manufactured in the plasma cells. The albumin fraction, fibrinogen and prothrombin are manufactured in the liver.

13 A False
  B True
  C True
  D False
  E True

Normal red cells are biconcave discs with a diameter of $7\,\mu$m. They circulate in the blood for 120 days. Red cell metabolism changes as the cell matures. The supply of energy to RBCs in the form of ATP is glycolysis with lactate production.

14 A False
  B True
  C True
  D True
  E True

Molecular weight of normal plasma albumin is 69 000 and the molecular weight of lipid-carrying β-globulins may be over 1 000 000

8 Acid/base

1 Hyponatraemia
A Occurs in patients with biliary fistulas
B Is aggravated by water excess
C Mean corpuscular volume is low and the haematocrit is high
D Serum potassium is high
E Can lead to a high pulse pressure

2 Anion gap
A Measures the residual anions in the body
B Normal anion gap is 9 mEq./l or less
C An increased anion gap is seen in hypokalaemia
D Is decreased in haemodilution
E Is decreased in hypoalbuminaemia

3 Acid/base balance
A Standard bicarbonate is the bicarbonate concentration in the plasma which is obtained at body temperature
B Normal standard bicarbonate value is 22–26 mEq./l
C Base excess is defined as the presence of an excess of base or a deficit of base in the blood
D Base excess can be determined from the Siggard–Andersen nomogram
E The amount of acid (mEq.) required to correct a metabolic alkalosis is calculated as body weight (kg) × 0.3 × base excess

Acid/base: Answers

1   A   True
     B   True
     C   False
     D   True
     E   False

Hyponatraemia is also seen in patients with vomiting, dysentery and small bowel obstruction. As the water enters the RBCs the haematocrit and the mean corpuscular volume are increased. Serum potassium and sodium concentrations vary in opposite directions, the cause being unknown. Owing to diminished blood volume, there may be orthostatic hypotension, low pulse pressure and tachycardia with a collapsing pulse.

2   A   True
     B   False
     C   True
     D   False
     E   True

Anion gap is usually the sum of measured cations (Na, K, Ca) which will be greater than the sum of anions (HCO_3, Cl), as other anions such as phosphates, sulphates and organic acids are not measured. The normal value for the anion gap is 16 mEq./l. In patients with water excess, the Na/K concentration can decrease by 10–20%, thus causing an increase in the anion gap. A decrease of 1 g of albumin/100 ml decreases the anion gap by 2.7 mEq./l.

3   A   False
     B   True
     C   True
     D   True
     E   True

Standard bicarbonate is the amount present in the plasma which is equilibrated at a PCO_2 of 40 mmHg, haemoglobin of 15 g fully saturated with oxygen at 37°C. Base excess is zero with a pH of 7.4 at a PCO_2 of 40 mmHg. A positive value indicates an excess of base (or a deficit of fixed acid).

4 Chemical buffers in the body
   A   Bicarbonate–carbonic acid buffer system operates in the intracellular water
   B   Phosphate buffer system functions in the kidney tubules
   C   Protein buffer system functions in the liver
   D   20% of carbon dioxide is transported in the RBCs as a carbamino compound with haemoglobin
   E   Sodium chloride has a strong neutralizing power

5 Acid/base balance
   A CO_2 content measures the total CO_2 which is liberated by the acidification of the plasma
   B   An uncompensated respiratory acidosis is characterized by a low pH, high PCO_2 and a low CO_2 content
   C   In uncompensated metabolic alkalosis there is a high pH, a normal PCO_2 and a high CO_2 content
   D   In a compensated metabolic acidosis the pH is normal, PO_2 becomes low and the CO_2 content rises
   E   In a compensated respiratory alkalosis, pH returns to normal, CO_2 content and the PCO_2 become low

6 Acid/base status
   A   In respiratory acidosis, ratio of HCO_3/PCO_2 is increased
   B   Standard bicarbonate is the amount of bicarbonate present when the blood is equilibrated at PCO_2 of 40 mmHg at 37°C when oxygen is fully saturated
   C   In respiratory alkalosis there is a negative base excess
   D   In metabolic alkalosis the pH is raised
   E   In metabolic acidosis the standard bicarbonate is low

4 A False
  B True
  C False
  D True
  E False

'Buffer' is a chemical substance which by its availability decreases the pH change caused by the addition of an acid or a base. A 'buffer' is a mixture of either a weak acid and its alkali salt or a weak base and its acid salt. Bicarbonate–carbonic acid buffer system is the largest component in the extracellular water. The protein buffer system is predominantly seen in the tissue cells and in the plasma.

5 A True
  B False
  C True
  D False
  E True

CO_2 content is the sum total of CO_2 dissolved in the plasma, CO_2 derived from bicarbonate and the CO_2 derived from plasma carbonic acid. CO_2 measurement is valuable in differential diagnosis. For example, if a diuretic is producing metabolic alkalosis it will be reflected as a rise in CO_2 content and a fall in serum potassium and chloride concentration. In an uncompensated respiratory acidosis there is a low pH, high P_{CO_2} and CO_2 content which changes to normal pH and an unchanged P_{CO_2} with a rising CO_2 content when compensated by a metabolic alkalosis. In a compensated metabolic acidosis the pH is normal and the P_{CO_2} and CO_2 content become low.

6 A False
  B True
  C True
  D True
  E True

An increase in P_{CO_2} reduces the HCO_3/P_{CO_2} ratio.

7 **Hypokalaemia**
   A   Urine is acidic
   B   Osmolality of urine rises
   C   Is seen in patients with thyroid malignancy
   D   Hyperglycaemia can be seen
   E   Prominent U waves are seen in the ECG in the left heart leads

8 **The following biochemical changes are seen in diabetic acidosis:**
   A   Low serum bicarbonate
   B   High serum sodium initially
   C   Elevated blood urea nitrogen
   D   Actual bicarbonate is higher than standard bicarbonate
   E   Anion gap is decreased

9 **Causes of hyperkalaemia**
   A   Addison's disease
   B   Frusemide
   C   Transfusion of stored bank blood
   D   Use of pancuronium
   E   Thrombocytosis

7 A True
   B False
   C True
   D True
   E False
In hypokalaemia, in the distal tubules, hydrogen ions are exchanged for potassium ions and excreted in the urine. The osmolality of the urine increases due to the inability of the kidneys to concentrate urine (hyposthenuria). In patients with medullary carcinoma of thyroid, the cancer cells produce prostaglandins which in turn cause diarrhoea and hypokalaemia by stimulating intestinal secretions. Low potassium levels cause decreased glucose tolerance, and prominent U waves are seen in the precordial leads V1–V4 of the ECG.

8 A True
   B False
   C True
   D False
   E False
The serum sodium is low because of sodium loss or the increased osmolality of the extracellular water caused by glucose. Actual bicarbonate is lower than standard bicarbonate indicating metabolic acidosis compensated by respiratory alkalosis. The anion gap is increased due to the production of lactic acid.

9 A True
   B False
   C True
   D False
   E True
Potassium-sparing diuretics, such as triamterene and spironolactone, and depolarizing muscle relaxants, such as suxamethonium, can contribute towards hyperkalaemia. Stored blood may contain about 20 mEq. of potassium ions/l if it is more than 10 days old.

10 Bicarbonates
   A When the standard bicarbonate is lower than actual bicarbonate it indicates respiratory acidosis
   B In metabolic acidosis standard bicarbonate is high
   C In an uncompensated metabolic acidosis both actual and standard bicarbonate are high and equal
   D The actual and standard bicarbonate values can vary by $+2\,mEq./l$
   E Actual and standard bicarbonate values can be derived from the Siggard–Andersen nomogram

11 In patients with uretero-enterostomy
   A Hyperchloraemic metabolic alkalosis is seen
   B Serum potassium is high
   C Large volume of water is excreted
   D Kussmaul breathing can be seen
   E Marked muscular weakness can be seen

12 Acid/base imbalance
   A Simultaneous respiratory and metabolic acidosis can be seen in a patient with cor-pulmonale on diuretic therapy
   B Simultaneous metabolic acidosis and respiratory alkalosis can be seen in patients with salicylate poisoning
   C Simultaneous respiratory and metabolic acidosis does not occur frequently
   D Diabetics may show a picture of metabolic alkalosis and metabolic acidosis
   E Respiratory alkalosis and metabolic alkalosis can be produced experimentally

10 A True
    B False
    C False
    D True
    E True
Under ideal conditions, standard bicarbonate and actual bicarbonate are equal. Astrup and co-workers showed that CO_2 capacity is similar to standrad bicarbonate and the CO_2 content is similar to actual bicarbonate. In an uncompensated metabolic acidosis, both actual and standard bicarbonate are low and equal.

11 A False
    B False
    C True
    D True
    E True
In this condition the patient suffers from hyperchloraemic metabolic acidosis. The serum potassium is low due to loss resulting from colonic secretion of potassium ions into the urine. A large volume of urine is excreted due to a continued re-excretion of sodium chloride and urea. Marked muscular weakness is seen due to low potassium.

12 A False
    B True
    C True
    D True
    E True
Respiratory acidosis with a metabolic alkalosis is seen in patients with cor-pulmonale (high standard bicarbonate, actual bicarbonate and CO_2 content). The picture in salicylate poisoning may comprise of normal pH, low P_{CO_2} (respiratory alkalosis), low CO_2 content and actual bicarbonate (metabolic acidosis). Simultaneous respiratory and metabolic acidosis can be produced experimentally by adding CO_2 to a ventilated patient whose heart failure is treated with ammonium chloride. If a diabetic starts vomiting he will develop metabolic alkalosis. Simultaneous respiratory and metabolic alkalosis can be produced experimentally by asking the patient to ingest sodium bicarbonate (producing metabolic alkalosis) and then asking him to hyperventilate (respiratory alkalosis).

13 **Metabolic alkalosis**
   A   Is seen with loop diuretics
   B   Is seen in hypocalcaemia
   C   Occurs in malignant hypertension
   D   Is seen in the anuric phase of acute renal failure
   E   Chloride concentration is low

14 **Inappropriate antidiuretic hormone secretion (IADH)**
   A   Serum osmolality is high
   B   Urine is hypotonic
   C   Clinical condition can be improved by fluid restriction
   D   Is a form of dilutional hyponatraemia
   E   Can be due to treatment with chlorpropamide

15 **Hyperchloraemic metabolic acidosis occurs in:**
   A   Diabetic ketoacidosis
   B   Diarrhoea
   C   Distal renal tubular acidosis
   D   Ethyl alcohol ketoacidosis
   E   Uretero-enterostomy

13 A True
B False
C True
D False
E True
With loop diuretics, hydrogen and chloride ions are low. In hypercalcaemia potassium is lost in the urine, hence metabolic alkalosis is seen in these conditions. Again, in the diuretic phase of renal failure, potassium loss in the urine causes metabolic alkalosis.

14 A False
B False
C True
D True
E True
In IADH syndrome the serum osmolality is low along with the serum sodium concentration. The urine is hypertonic as the plasma is diluted with water and the urine contains an adequate amount of sodium ions. Chlorpropamide produces IADH by potentiating the action of ADH on the kidneys, although it may stimulate ADH secretion centrally.

15 A False
B True
C True
D False
E True
In diabetic ketoacidosis and ethyl alcohol ketoacidosis, the chloride levels are normal.

16 Water intoxication
  A   Is seen in acute bronchopneumonia
  B   Occurs in Cushing's syndrome
  C   Can occur following vomiting
  D   Normally, when the volume of extracellular water rises, aldosterone secretion is increased
  E   Convulsions can occur

17 Lactic acidosis is seen in:
  A   Acute pulmonary oedema
  B   Acute pyelonephritis
  C   Cardiopulmonary bypass
  D   Acute leukaemia
  E   Phenformin treatment of diabetes mellitus

16 A True
B False
C True
D False
E True

Water intoxication is seen in bronchopneumonia due to excess ADH secretion. It is also seen in Addison's disease. Following vomiting, sodium loss occurs causing a fall in osmotic pressure of blood and extracellular fluid (ECF) as compared with the cells, thus allowing water from the former to enter the cells causing them to swell.

17 A True
B True
C True
D True
E True

Lactic acidosis occurs during the hypothermic phase of cardiopulmonary bypass. Lactic acid is formed by the white blood cells in leukaemia and the cause is unknown in acute pyelonephritis.

9 Statistics

1 Statistics

A Standard error of the mean is defined as the standard deviations divided by the number of observations

B Null hypothesis demonstrates that there is no difference between the two-sample tests

C Student's 't' test is used for large samples

D Chi square test is used for measuring differences in derived statistics

E Chi square test is the sum of observed minus expected results squared divided by the expected results

2 Statistical tests

A Paired 't' test (parametric) can be substituted by Wilcoxon rank sum test

B Two-sample 't' test has no substitute non-parametric test

C Spearmans' rank correlation coefficient is an alternative to product moment correlation coefficient (a parametric test)

D Mann–Whitney U test is a distribution-free test

E Wilcoxon rank sum test compares the distributions of observations in two populations

3 Statistical definitions

A Frequencies or scores which have no fixed numerical value are non-parametric

B Numerical characteristics of a given population are called parameters

C A curve with a concave top and convex tails on either side is called a normal distribution curve

D Mode = mean − 2 (mean − median)

E Mean value is the sum of values divided by the number of observations

Statistics: Answers

1   A   False
    B   True
    C   False
    D   False
    E   True
Standard error of mean (S.E.M.) is the standard deviation divided by the square root of the number of observations. Student's 't' test is used to measure samples less than 60. Chi square test is used to measure changes in actual numbers of occurrences and not percentages or other derived statistics.

2   A   False
    B   False
    C   True
    D   True
    E   True
Wilcoxon signed rank test (a non-parametric test) can substitute for the paired 't' test. Similarly, Wilcoxon rank sum test can replace the two-sample 't' test.

3   A   True
    B   True
    C   False
    D   False
    E   True
A curve with a convex top and concave tail is called normal or Gaussian distribution. Mode + mean − 3 (mean − median) is a normal relationship.

4 Tests of hypothesis
  A   Null hypothesis is formulated for the purpose of being rejected or nullified
  B   Type I error is a statistical hypothesis which is rejected when it is not true
  C   Type II error is a statistical hypothesis which is rejected when it is true
  D   Significance level is associated with a Type I error
  E   Critical region (rejection region) is a set of values of the test leading to rejection of null hypothesis

5 Statistics
  A   Wilcoxon rank sum test is a highly sensitive test as compared with the Student's 't' test
  B   Chi square test is useful in testing the presence or absence of association between characteristics which cannot be quantitatively expressed
  C   The distribution of 't' was worked out by Gosset in 1908
  D   't' test compares two means and sees how much they depart from the standard deviation of these two means
  E   Standard error of mean is the product of standard deviations divided by the number of observations

6 Abbreviations used in statistics
  A   S.E.M. is the standard error of mode
  B r is the correlation coefficient
  C $n - 1$ is the number of observations in a sample
  D SS is the sum of squared deviations from the mean
  E S is the estimate of population variance based on sample statistics

7 Linear regression
  A   Is an independent relationship between one variable to another variable
  B y is the random variable
  C x is a variable which is used to predict y
  D   Alpha (α) is the value of x when $y = 0$
  E   Beta (β) is a gradient which measures the slope of the line

4 A True
   B False
   C False
   D True
   E True

Type I error is a statistical hypothesis which is rejected when it is true and Type II error is a hypothesis which is not rejected when it is not false.

5 A False
   B True
   C True
   D False
   E False

The 't' test is a more sensitive test for genuine difference than the Rank test which is also applicable for paired observations. Gosset in 1908 wrote the distribution of 't' under the pseudonym of 'Student', which later on came to be known as Student's 't' test.

The 't' test = Difference between two means/Standard error of that difference

Similarly, standard error of mean = Standard deviation/Square root of the number of observations

6 A False
   B True
   C False
   D True
   E True

S.E.M. is the standard error of the mean and $n - 1$ is the degree of freedom, i.e. number of observations minus one.

7 A False
   B True
   C True
   D False
   E True

Linear regression is based on the dependence of one variable x on the other variable y. y is a dependent variable in a linear regression line. $y = $ alpha (α) + beta (β) x. x is an independent variable capable of measurement without an error. Alpha (α) is a parameter called the intercept of the line and is the value of $y = 0$. Beta (β) is also called the regression coefficient which measures the slope of the line, i.e. the change in y per unit increase in x.

8 Statistics
- A Coefficient of variation is the standard deviation of the distribution expressed as a percentage of the mean of the distribution
- B 95.45% of the observations lie within +3 times the standard deviation from the mean
- C 68.27% proportion of observations lie within +1 times the standard deviation from the mean
- D In an ideal normal frequency distribution, the mean, mode and median all coincide
- E Normal frequency distribution curve becomes concave around the mean

9 Descriptive statistics
- A Median is the middle of the range observation
- B Mode is the most commonly occurring value
- C Range is the dispersion between the largest and the smallest value
- D Standard deviation is a measure of the differences of each observation from the mean
- E Variance is the mean squared deviation

10 Correlation coefficient
- A Relates to the interdependence between the two variables x and y
- B $r = 0$ indicates a non-linear relationship
- C $r = +0$ indicates a perfect correlation
- D $r = -1$ indicates a perfect positive correlation
- E $r = +1$ is a perfect negative correlation

8 A True
   B False
   C True
   D True
   E False
The coefficient of variation is (standard deviation/mean) x 100.
95.45% of the observations lie within 2 standard deviations and at 3
it is 99.73%. The normal frequency distribution curve is symmetrical
around the mean.

9 A False
   B True
   C False
   D True
   E True
Median is the value of the middle observation when they are
arranged in order of size. Range is the difference between the two
values. Variance is derived by squaring all the deviations from the
mean followed by dividing them with the number in the sample.

10 A True
    B True
    C False
    D False
    E False
Correlation coefficient is represented by the letter r. The magnitude
of r indicates the strength of the linear relationship between x and
y. $r = +1$ indicates that all the points lie on the line. $r = +1$ is a
perfect positive correlation in which as x increases, y increases.

Bibliography

The multiple choice questions were compiled with the guidance of the following textbooks and journals.

(1) Gannong, W.F. (ed.) (1989) *Review of Medical Physiology*
(2) Scurr, C., Feldman, S. and Soni, N. (eds.) (1990) *Scientific Foundations of Anaesthesia*
(3) Nunn, J.F. (ed.) (1978) *Applied Respiratory Physiology*
(4) Baron, D.N. (ed.) (1979) *A Short Textbook of Chemical Pathology*
(5) Hewer, C.L. and Atkinson, R.S. (eds) (1979) *Recent Advances in Anaesthesia and Analgesia*, No. 13
(6) Atkinson, R.S. (ed.) (1982) *Recent Advances in Anaesthesia and Analgesia*, No. 14
(7) Atkinson, R.S. and Adams, A.P. (eds) (1985) *Recent Advances in Anaesthesia and Analgesia*, No. 15
(8) West, J.B. (ed.) (1987) *Respiratory Physiology*
(9) Sykes, M.K., McNicol, M.W. and Campbell, E.J.M. (eds) (1976) *Respiratory Failure*
(10) Guyton, A.C. (ed.) (1984) *Physiology of the Human Body*
(11) Petrie, A. (ed.) (1980) *Lecture Notes on Medical Statistics*
(12) Swinscow, T.D.V. (ed.) (1974) *Statistics at Square One*
(13) Hill, A.B. (ed.) (1977) *A Short Textbook of Medical Statistics*
(14) Goldberger, E. (ed.) (1980) *A Primer of Water, Electrolyte and Acid Base Syndromes*
(15) Laurence, D.R. and Bennett, P.N. (eds) (1987) *Clinical Pharmacology*
(16) Vickers, M.D., Wood-Smith, F.G. and Stewart, H.C. (eds) (1990) *Drugs in Anaesthetic Practice*
(17) Meyers, F.H., Jawetz, E. and Goldfien, A. (eds) (1987) *Review of Medical Pharmacology*
(18) Moir, D.D. (ed.) (1980) *Obstetric Anaesthesia and Analgesia*
(19) *The Clinical Use of Ranitidine. A Glaxo International Symposium*
(20) *Hypnovel in Anaesthesia*, Roche
(21) *Isoflurane. Abstracts from VIII World Congress of Anaesthesiologists*, Manila
(22) Propofol Symposium, *Postgraduate Medical Journal*
(23) Best, J.B. and Taylor, S. (eds) (1987) *Physiological Basis of Medical Practice*
(24) Goodman, L.S. and Gilman, A. (eds) (1987) *Pharmacological Basis of Therapeutics*
(25) *Anaesthesia and Analgesia* (1987) **15**, 1–43

Bibliography

(26) *British Journal of Anaesthesia* (1987) **59** 14–23
(27) Wood, M. and Wood, A. (eds) (1990) *Drugs and Anesthesia*
(28) Stoetling (1987) *Pharmacology and Physiology in Anesthetic Practice*
(29) Heijke, S. and Smith, G. (1990) Quest for the ideal inhalation anaesthetic agent. Editorial *British Journal of Anaesthesia*
(30) Sasada, M.P. and Smith, S.P. (1990) *Drugs in Anaesthesia and Intensive Care*
(31) Dundee, J., Clarke, R.S. and McCaughey, W. (1991) *Clinical Anaesthetic Pharmacology*
(32) Wingard, Brody, Larner and Schwartz, (1991) *Human Pharmacology*

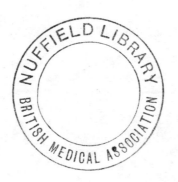